Medical Basics

A Self-Instructional Text

Anatomy

Normal Function

Common Injury

Common Disease

Medical Terms

Terminology

ICD-9 Codes

Linda Gifford-Meuleveld, R.N., C.O.H.N.-S.

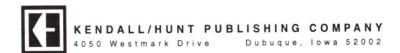
KENDALL/HUNT PUBLISHING COMPANY
4050 Westmark Drive   Dubuque, Iowa 52002

Medical Basics   Table of Contents

Preface

This book is useful for anyone that needs to apply a knowledge of medical basics in the workplace.

It is specifically designed to increase knowledge. It focuses on the anatomy of the working adult, while discussing normal function, common injury and disease. Medical terms, terminology and ICD-9* codes are included.

Originally, it was developed to train employees working with workers' compensation claims to have improved decision making ability. It was successful, and it's scope of application widened as it was discovered by others outside the insurance world.

Numerous professional organizations have found this information valuable, and have granted continuing education credits to individuals completing the course of study. In the last few years it has been used to fill a training need for:

- vocational coordinators

- legal assistants

- medical office workers

- radiological technicians

- safety officers

- occupational health nurses

- medical transcriptionists

- medical billing specialists

The strength of the book is that it is easily understood, communicating information that can readily be applied in the work world.

* ICD-9 (International Classification of Diseases, 9th revision) codes provide numerical coding of diseases, injuries, and procedures. They are used for billing medical services.

Many of the ICD-9 codes included in this text were determined to be among those frequently seen in medical billings for injured workers.

Acknowledgments

This text presents the shared output of several authors. Much of the information was compiled through collegial editing of my original text, with each successive person adding and deleting text, until the final content was achieved. I would like to thank many of the staff at SAIF corporation for their contribution, including:

Diane Firsich, RN, BSN, Medical Programs Manager,

Kathleen Cellucci, RN, BSN, COHN-S, Nurse Consultant

Pam Call, RN, BSN, Nurse Consultant, Case Manager

Carol Martin, RN, COHN-S, Nurse Reviewer

Ann Grim, Copy Editor

Lisa Taaffe, Graphic Design Coordinator

Kathleen Roberts, Graphics Designer

David Smith, Claims Adjuster

The final work was edited for accuracy of it's medical content by Robert Strukel, M.D..

Medical illustrations were supplied by LifeArt Images, TechPool Studios, Inc.

Introduction

Welcome to Medical Basics!

This book was developed to help you learn more about the medical aspects of injury in the working adult.

Using my experience as a hospital nurse, occupational health nurse, nurse consultant and medical trainer, I pulled together the information I felt you should know.

As you work your way through the book, you will find that some topics receive more attention than others. I have tried to create a balance of information that will be most useful to you in terms of overall application.

Medical Basics

Chapter 1

Medical Terminology: Learning the ABC's

Medical words can look formidable and intimidating.
Decoding these words is the first step to understanding them.

FIRST: Look at the word and analyze it's structure. Each word can be divided into it's basic components. The components are roots, suffixes, and prefixes. These can be called the ABC's of medical terminology:

A. ROOTS…usually indicate the body part affected by a condition:

Arth, Arthr, arthro ....joint
Ceph, or cephal ....head — cRanis —
Osteo ....bone
Chondri, chondro ....cartilage
My or myo ....muscle
Neur ....nerve
Cardi ....heart
Spondyl, spondylo *Spondelo* ....vertebra
Gaster, gastero, gastro ....stomach
Hem, hemato..............................blood
Dermis   *Skin*

B. SUFFIXES…are found at the end of a word:

algia, or algesia ....pain, suffering
pathy ....a disease or abnormal condition
itis ....inflammation
plasty..form or reform
otomy ....a surgical incision, cutting into
ectomy ....cutting out by surgical procedure
osis ....condition, disease
asthenia ....weakness, loss of strength
lysis ....freeing of
olisthesis ....slipping
malacia ....softening
oma ....tumor or clot

C. PREFIXES…are found at the beginning of a word:

Hyper ....above normal, excessive
Hypo ....less than normal, below, under
En ....in
Epi...on, upon
Para ....alongside, near
Peri ....around
Sub ....under
supra ....over, above
poly ....many
inter ....between

3

Can you use this process to decode the following words?

C 1. Arthritis: Joint inflamation

C 2. Cephalgia: head pain - suffering

C 3. Osteoarthritis: Bone joint inflamation

C 4. Osteochondritis: Bone Cartilage Inflamation

C 5. Myopathy: muscle disease

C 6. Neurasthenia: nerve weakness, loss of strength

C 7. Pericarditis: around heart inflamation

C 8. Spondylitis: vertabra inflamation

C 9. Spondylolisthesis: Vertabra Slipping

C 10. Gastritis: Stomach Inflamation

C 11. Chondromalacia: Cartilage softening

C 12. Encephalitis: In head inflamation

C 13. Neurosis: nerve condition

C 14. Polyneuritis: many nerve inflamation

C 15. Neurolysis: nerve freeing of

C 16. Subpericardial: under around heart

C 17. Osteotomy: bone surgical incision

C 18. Intervertebral: between vertebra

C 19. Cardiopathy: heart disease

C 20. Neuritis: nerve inflamation

C 21. Neuralgia: nerve pain

C 22. Hematoma: blood tumor

C 23. Epigastric: upon stomach

C 24. Gastroplasty: Stomach form

Answers:

1.	Arthritis:	joint...inflammation
2.	Cephalgia:	head...pain (headache)
3.	Osteoarthritis:	bone...joint...inflammation
4.	Osteochondritis:	bone...cartilage...inflammation
5.	Myopathy:	muscle...disease or abnormal condition of
6.	Neurasthenia:	nerve...weakness, loss of strength
7.	Pericarditis:	around...the heart...inflammation
8.	Spondylitis:	vertebra...inflammation
9.	Spondylolisthesis:	vertebra...slipping
10.	Gastritis:	stomach...inflammation
11.	Chondromalacia:	cartilage...softening
12.	Encephalitis:	in...head...inflammation
13.	Neurosis:	nerve...condition, disease
14.	Polyneuritis:	many...nerve...inflammation of
15.	Neurolysis:	nerve...freeing of
16.	Subpericardial:	under...around...heart
17.	Osteotomy:	bone...cutting into, surgical incision
18.	Intervertebral:	between...vertebra
19.	Cardiopathy:	heart...disease, abnormal condition
20.	Neuritis:	nerve...inflammation
21.	Neuralgia:	nerve...pain, suffering
22.	Hematoma:	blood...tumor, clot
23.	Epigastric:	on, upon...stomach
24.	Gastroplasty:	stomach...form, reform

MEDICAL TERMINOLOGY   Roots...Suffixes...Prefixes

ab, ac	AWAY FROM	ABDUCT/ACCIDENT
ad, af	TO	ADDUCT/AFFERENT
ante	BEFORE	ANTEFLEXION
anti	AGAINST	ANTIINFLAMITORY
arthr	JOINT	ARTHRITIS
articul	JOINT	DISARTICULATE
bi	TWO	BIVALVE
brachi	ARM	BRACHIOPLEXUS
brandy	SLOW	BRADYCARDIA
cardi	HEART	CARDIAC
caud	TAIL	CAUDA EQUINUS
cephal	HEAD	HYDROCEPHALIC
chondr	CARTILAGE	CHONDROMALACIA
circum	AROUND	CIRCUMFERENCE
co, con	WITH/TOGETHER	COHESION/CONTRACTION
contra	AGAINST/COUNTER	CONTRAINDICATED
crani	SKULL	CRANIUM
cyst	BLADDER	CYSTITIS
cut	SKIN	SUBCUTANEOUS
derm	SKIN	DERMATITIS
di	TWO	DISSECT
digit	FINGER/TOE	DIGIT
disc	DISK	DISCECTOMY
dors	BACK	DORSAL

MEDICAL TERMINOLOGY

Roots...Suffixes...Prefixes

dys	BAD/IMPROPER	**DYS**TROPHY
ex	OUT OF	**EX**CRETION
extra	OUTSIDE OF/BEYOND	**EXTRA**CELLULAR
febr	FEVER	A**FEBR**ILE
fract	BREAK	**FRACT**URE
gangli	SWELLING/PLEXUS	**GANGLI**ON CYST
gram	WRITE/RECORD	MYELO**GRAM**
hem	BLOOD	**HEM**ATOLOGY
hemi	HALF	**HEMI**SPHERE
hom, homo	COMMON/SAME	**HOMO**MORPHIC
hyper	ABOVE/BEYOND	**HYPER**TROPHY
hypo	UNDER/BELOW	**HYPO**THERMIA
infra	BELOW	**INFRA**ORBITAL
inter	AMONG/BETWEEN	**INTER**VERTEBRAL
intra	INSIDE	**INTRA**VENOUS
itis	INFl AMMATION	FASC**ITIS**/ARTHR**ITIS**
lith	STONE	**LITH**OTOMY
mal	BAD/ABNORMAL	**MAL**FUNCTION
medi	MIDDLE	**MEDI**ASTINAL
mega	LARGE	ACRO**MEGA**LY
meta	AFTER/BEYOND	**META**CARPAL
my	MUSCLE	**MY**OSITIS
ortho	STRAIGHT/NORMAL	**ORTHO**PEDICS
oss, ost	BONE	**OST**EOARTHRITIS
path	SICKNESS	**PATH**OLOGIST

MEDICAL TERMINOLOGY

Roots…Suffixes…Prefixes

peri	AROUND	**PERI**CARDITIS
phleb	VEIN	**PHLEB**ITIS
pneum	BREATH/AIR	**PNEUM**ONIA
pod	FOOT	**POD**IATRIST
post	AFTER/BEHIND	**POST**ERIOR
pre	BEFORE	**PRE**DISPOSED
psych	SOUL/MIND	**PSYCH**OSOCIAL
pulmo	LUNG	**PULMO**NARY
quadr	FOUR	**QUADR**ICEPS
retro	BACKWARDS	**RETRO**GRADE FEVER
rub	RED	**RUB**RA COLOR
semi	HALF	**SEMI**FLEXION
sep	ROT/DECAY	**SEP**SIS
somat	BODY	PSYCHOS**OMAT**IC
spas	DRAW/PULL	**SPAS**M
staphyl	BUNCH OF GRAPES	**STAPHYL**OCOCCUS
strep	TWIST	**STREP**TOCOCCUS
sub	UNDER/BELOW	**SUB**CONSCIOUS
therap	TREATMENT	HYDRO**THERAP**Y
therm	HEAT	**THERM**OGRAPHY
thorac	CHEST	**THORAC**IC
thromb	LUMP/CLOT	**THROMB**OPHLEBITIS
tri	THREE	**TRI**GEMINAL
tuber	SWELLING/NODE	**TUBER**CLE
un	ONE	**UN**ILATERAL
zo	LIFE	**ZO**OLOGY

TOPIC: SKULL   (Crani...root word for skull)

1. **There are 8 cranial bones: FRONTAL (1), PARIETAL (2), OCCIPITAL (1), TEMPORAL (2), SPHENOID (2), ETHMOID (1)**

   These bones are firmly interlocked along irregular lines called sutures.
   They combine to form the cranium. The cranium encloses the brain.

2. **There are 13 facial bones forming the facial skeleton.**

3. **The MANDIBLE is one bone. It forms the lower jaw. It is a movable bone held to the cranium by ligaments.**

4. **Skull fractures are the most common injury to the skull. A FRACTURE is the sudden breaking of a bone.**

SIMPLE Fracture:	a bone is broken, but there is no open wound in the skin. (also called a closed fracture)
COMPOUND Fracture:	a broken bone with an open wound in the skin. (also called an open fracture)

5. **Common types of skull fractures are:**

LINEAR:	a simple crack of the bone. The bone is not fragmented into pieces.
COMMINUTED:	A bone is splintered or crushed into more than two pieces.
DEPRESSED:	A piece of the broken bone is driven inward and presses on the brain.
BASAL:	The lower part of the skull, on which the brain rests. This is a common site for fractures. It is the most common, and potentially the most dangerous type of skull fracture. The danger exists because the basal skull area is in close proximity to the cranial nerves, major blood vessels, and nerve centers.

6. **ICD-9:ICD-9 codes commonly seen for injured workers with skull injury are:**

800.00	Fractured skull, Vault closed...includes frontal and parietal bones
801.50	Fractured skull, Base open...includes occiput bone, orbital roof, sinus, ethmoid, temporal, sphenoid bone

7. **The major function of the skull is protection of the brain.**

TOPIC: BRAIN   (encephal…root word for brain)
(cephal…root word for head)

The brain is the body's control center. It is linked to the rest of the body by nerves. The nerves send messages to the brain by electric current. The brain weighs approximately 3 pounds, and contains about 14 billion nerve cells. These nerve cells are responsible for decoding the electrical impulses received by the brain.

1. **The MENINGES are three soft layers of tissue that cover the brain. These three protective layers of membrane surround the brain and spinal cord. Moving from brain to skull, the three layers are identified as:**

    Pia mater ……………closest to brain

    Arachnoid……………the middle membrane

    Dura mater …………closest to the skull

2. **The brain and it's coverings fit snugly inside the skull. A skull fracture is an injury to the skull that can cause bleeding. There is no room for the clotted blood, and the rigid skull cannot expand. The pressure is then exerted on the soft brain tissue and it's coverings. The blood clot is called a HEMATOMA.**

    EPIDURAL HEMATOMA ………a blood clot on or above the dura mater.

    SUBDURAL HEMATOMA ………a blood clot under the dura mater
    A epidural hematoma can be very serious. Bleeding is forceful, coming from the arteries, creating large clots. Pressure from a epidural hematoma can cause rapid death if surgery is not done quickly.

    A subdural hematoma creates problems more slowly, due to the slower bleeding from smaller veins. Surgery, however, is usually necessary to remove the clot.

3. **A CEREBRAL HEMORRHAGE** is a hemorrhage (of blood) in the brain or it's coverings. It is the cause of a cerebral hematoma.

4. **BRAIN CONTUSION:** an injury that bruises the brain, but does not tear the brain or it's coverings. A slight bruise will create mild swelling, and mild symptoms..such as a brief "black-out". A severe bruise will create severe swelling. The injury will cause symptoms corresponding to the amount of pressure on the brain. The most severe complication of a contusion is death.

5. **BRAIN LACERATION:** A serious injury that tears into the brain. It is usually accompanied by a depressed skull fracture. Nerve impairment is probable.

TOPIC: BRAIN (Continued)

6. **BRAIN CONCUSSION:** An injury in which the brain is violently shaken. Immediate symptoms can include a brief loss of consciousness, temporary dizziness, disorientation, or sudden vomiting. Residual symptoms of headache, nervousness, dizziness, ringing in the ears and blurred vision can persist for a while after the initial injury. Most commonly occurs in males between the ages of 19-35. They are often concussions in the mild to severe range.

7. **CEPHALGIA:** A medical term for headache. (cephal=head, algia=pain)

8. **SEIZURE:** A sudden episode of uncontrolled electrical activity in the brain. If the electrical activity spreads throughout the brain, consciousness is lost, and a grand mal seizure results. Recurrent seizures are called **EPILEPSY**. There can be many causes for seizures, including head injury, infection, and stroke.

9. **CVA:** A cerebrovascular accident, commonly called a stroke. It usually occurs within the cerebrum, the largest part of the brain. The brain is damaged by either ischemia or a hemorrhage.

    ISCHEMIA...insufficient blood supply due to some form of obstruction of blood flow. The obstruction can be in the form of a blood clot or embolism. (T.I.A. - Transient Ischemic Attack)

    HEMORRHAGE...abnormal discharge of blood (into the tissues of the brain.)

10. **COMA:** A state of unconsciousness in which the person cannot be aroused. 50% of all comas are either the result of a CVA or head trauma.

    Irreversible coma indicates that the brain has stopped normal function.

11. **ICD-9 codes commonly seen for injured workers with brain injury:**

    853.09 ....Hematoma w/ Concussion

    784.0 ....Headache

    345.5 ....Epilepsy

12. **DISABILITY:** Severe trauma to the head can lead to damage of the brain. At time of closure, solicit the class of impairment from the physician. OAR 436-35-390

TOPIC: THE CRANIAL NERVES

1. **Twelve pairs of cranial nerves emerge from the base of the brain.** They are usually identified by Roman numerals I through XII. The cranial nerves carry impulses between the brain and the head and neck.

2. **The consequences of cranial nerve injuries depend on the location and extent of the injuries.** For example, if only one member of a nerve pair is damaged, loss of function is limited to the affected side, but if both nerves are injured, losses occur on both sides. Also, if a nerve is severed completely, the functional loss is total; if the cut is incomplete, the loss may be partial.

3. **The tenth cranial nerve, the Vagus Nerve, is one of the most important components of the parasympathetic nervous system.** It helps maintain the rhythmic automatic function of the internal body machinery. It has branches to all the main digestive organs, the heart, and the lungs.

4. **TRIGEMINAL NEURALGIA:** A painful disorder of the 5th cranial nerve. It is also called Tic Douloureux. It is usually related to some form of compression of the nerve root, in the form of tumors or vascular lesions, but rarely trauma. Occassionally it can be related to an underlying condition of multiple sclerosis or herpes zoster.

5. **BELL'S PALSY:** A disease of the 7th cranial nerve that produces one sided facial weakness or paralysis. It is often associated with infections and can result from local trauma, hemorrhage, or tumor.

6. **ICD-9's and disability are directed to the body part innervated by the nerve that is injured.**

    350.1   ....trigiminal neuralgia

    351.0   ....Bell's palsy

7. **See cranial nerve chart for details of individual function.**

Cranial Nerve Chart

I.   Olfactory . . . . Related to the sense of smell

II.   Optic . . . . Related to the sense of sight

III.   Oculomotor . . . . . . Extends to the voluntary and involuntary muscles of the eye

IV.   Trochlear . . . . Smallest cranial nerve, goes to external eye muscles

V.   Trigeminal . . . . Largest cranial nerve, has three branches going to the face

VI.   Abducens . . . . Extends to external eye muscles

VII.   Facial . . . . Related to the production of tears and saliva

VIII.   Vestibulocochlear . . Related to hearing, sometimes called the auditory nerve

IX.   Glossopharyngeal . . Extends to the tongue and pharynx

X.   Vagus . . . . Extends down through the neck, chest and abdomen

XI.   Accessory . . . . Extends to the neck and upper back

XII.   Hypoglossal . . . . . Extends to the tongue, influences speaking, chewing, swallowing

Medical Basics

Chapter 1

Topic: THE EYE

(ocul…root word for eye)
(opthalm…root word for eye)
(blephar…root word for eyelid)

1. **The eye is the organ of sight.** It consists of structures that focus an image onto the retina at the back of the eye. In the retina, a network of nerves convert the image into electrical impulses recorded in a region of the brain…It works like a camera, only much faster. Both need light, and both have lenses to make the picture clear. The eye has no film, but it does have the retina. The retina is a tissue lining the back of the interior of the eye. It has special cells that are sensitive to light. There are approximately 132 million light sensitive cells in the retina of each eye. Messages from these cells travel from the retina, to the optic nerve, and on to the brain.

2. **The lens, cornea, retina, optic nerve, and conjunctiva are frequently mentioned in reports of injury to the eye. Identify each on the diagram of the eye.**

3. **Right eye, left eye and both eyes are commonly abbreviated:**

   O.D ....right eye

   O.S...left eye

   O.U ....both eyes, or sometimes used to designate either eye

4. **CORNEAL ABRASION:** A "scratch" on the cornea usually caused by a foreign body. It can be quite painful, with much tearing and sensitivity to light. It may be symptomatic for 24-48 hours.

5. **CONJUNCTIVITIS:** The membrane covering the eye becomes irritated. It can be caused by exposure of the eye to chemicals, dust, or smoke. It usually clears quickly with treatment, and has no permanent residual.

6. **CATARACT:** The lens of the eye becomes opaque, causing blurred vision. It may be caused by injury or naturally occurring degeneration due to aging. Injuries commonly causing cataracts are contusions to the eye, or penetration of the lens by small flying pieces of metal or wood. CATARACT REMOVAL means surgical removal of the lens. When this is done, a substitution must be made, to create the new lens. Corrective reading glasses or lenses will be an ongoing necessity.

7. **DIPLOPIA:** Double vision. It can be either a symptom or a condition, caused by injury or disease.

8. **NYSTAGMUS:** Involuntary, recurring eyeball movement. It produces blurred vision, and difficulty in focusing. It is sometimes congenital, but is most frequently results from head injury involving the ear, or from any inflammation of the brain (such as encephalitis or meningitis).

9. **STRABISMUS:** An observable deviation in the normal parallel alignment of the eyes. (such as "cross-eye")

Topic: THE EYE (Continued)

10. **ENUCLEATION:** Complete removal of the eye from it's socket, causing blindness.

11. **GLAUCOMA:** Swelling in the eye, which can damage the optic nerve. If untreated, it can lead to loss of vision. 90% of patients with glaucoma have a variety that is naturally occurring, familial in origin. Secondary glaucoma can result from trauma, inflammation, or drugs (such as steroids).

12. **RETINAL DETACHMENT:** The layers of the retina become separated, creating a subretinal space. The space fills with fluid. Symptoms may include recurrent flashes of light, progressing to a gradual, painless vision loss. The degenerative changes of age usually cause this problem. Trauma to the head or eye has been said to cause some occurrences. It is twice as common in men as women.

13. **DIABETIC RETINOPATHY:** When diabetes is poorly controlled, resulting in blood sugar levels higher than normal on an ongoing basis, it can harm the blood vessels in the eyes. Small vessels can rupture, causing vision loss. Close monitoring and control of blood sugar is linked to the progression of this disease. Diabetic retinopathy is a leading cause of acquired adult blindness. Laser treatment directed at sealing off the small ruptured blood vessels is sometimes beneficial.

14. **COLOR BLINDNESS:** the retina has cells called rods, these determine black and white. It also has cells called cones, that determine color. A person cannot see color because some of the cones are not working properly. If none are working, all colors are perceived as gray. This condition is called monochromasia.

15. **HOW DOES THE EYE ALLOW US TO SEE?:** Light enters through the dark center of the eye... the PUPIL. The CORNEA is a fibrous, transparent tissue that covers the pupil and the colored part of the eye. The function of the cornea is to bend ...or, REFRACT...rays of light so they can focus properly on the back of the eye. The IRIS helps regulate the amount of light allowed to enter the eye. The LENS helps bend the light rays that enter the eye. The RETINA is the sensitive nerve layer lining the interior of the eyeball. It converts the light rays to electrical impulses that are transferred to the OPTIC NERVE.

    The optic nerve leaves the eye ball, then before entering the brain, it crosses over...at the OPTIC CHIASM...and enters the brain on the opposite side of the head...the optic nerve from the right eye will enter the left side of the brain. The brain then decodes the electrical impulses.

16. **ICD Codes commonly seen for injured workers with eye injury:**

    918.1   ....Superficial Injury to the Cornea

    930.0   ....Foreign Body

    372.05 ....Conjunctivitis

TOPIC: THE EAR

(oto…root word for ear)

(aur…root word for ear)

1. **THE EAR CONSISTS OF THREE PARTS:** The outer ear, the middle ear, and the inner ear.

2. The outer and middle ear are concerned primarily with the collection and transmission of sound.

3. The inner ear is responsible for analyzing sound waves. It also contains the mechanism that helps the body keep it's balance.

4. The external portion of the ear collects and funnels sound waves to the eardrum. The eardrum separates the outer ear from the middle ear. It vibrates in response to the changes in air pressure that constitute sound. The ear drum vibrations are sent to the three small bones in the middle ear. They send the sound waves on to the nerve endings in the internal ear. This nerve is the auditory nerve. The nerve carries the message to the brain.

5. **Hearing impairment is classified as either conductive or perceptive.**

   CONDUCTIVE IMPAIRMENT: Usually due to a problem in the external or middle ear. Can be caused by ear wax, foreign bodies, or infection. It rarely results in complete deafness.

   PERCEPTIVE IMPAIRMENT: Is also called hearing nerve impairment. This can be caused by infection, extreme levels of noise, or reaction to chemicals. Hearing can be seriously impaired.

6. **EUSTACHIAN TUBE:** A small tube leading from the middle ear to the pharynx, in the upper throat. If it becomes plugged, otitis media can result.

7. **OTITIS MEDIA:** Inflammation of the middle ear. It is usually treated with antibiotic and decongestant medication.

8. **TINNITUS:** A ringing, buzzing, or whistling noise heard in the ear in the absence of environmental noise. It can be a symptom of a treatable ear disorder, such as otitis media. Occasionally there is no treatment other than masking the sound, by creating a diversionary sound.

9. **MENIERE'S DISEASE:** A recurrent and progressive group of symptoms that include progressive deafness, ringing in the ears, dizziness, and sometimes a sensation of fullness in the ears. It is treated with medication, and rarely surgery.

10. **LABYRINTH:** Another name for the internal ear. It is essential for maintaining physical equilibrium in the body. It is a complex system of sacks and tubes containing endolymph. Endolymph is a pale transparent fluid.

TOPIC: THE EAR   (Continued)

11. **BALANCE:** The vestibular nerve is a main division of the auditory nerve. It helps determine balance. The vestibular system is closely connected to the cochlea. Receptors in this system are sensitive to changes in movement of the endolymph. Balance comes from a combination of messages from the eyes, the vestibular system, and the nerve endings in muscles and joints. These nerve endings in muscles and joints are called **PROPRIOCEPTORS.** All of these things work in unison to provide a conscious appreciation of the position of the body.

12. **FOREIGN BODY:** Slivers, cinders, dirt, or small objects that lodge in the ears (skin, eyes, nose, or internally).

13. **DISABILITY:** In order to determine hearing loss impairment, the following is needed: an audiogram performed within six months of the medically stationary date. The audiogram must report on air conduction frequencies at 500, 1,000, 2,000, 3,000, 4,000 and 6,000 Hz. Hearing loss claims are processes internally here at SAIF, by the Disability Section.

14. **ICD-9 codes commonly seen for injured workers involving the ear:**

    389.10 ....Hearing loss

    931. ....Foreign body, ear

TOPIC: THE MOUTH AND JAW   (Dent…root word for tooth)
(Buccal…root word for mouth)
(OS…mouth)

1. **TONGUE:** The muscular, flexible organ that occupies the floor of the mouth. It is responsible for breaking down food as it passes through the mouth, as well as assisting in swallowing and speech.

2. **TEETH:** Hard, bony structures set in the jaw, that are used for mastication (chewing food). There are 32 permanent teeth, 16 on top and bottom.

   central incisor: ……………(4) two on top and two on the bottom

   lateral incisor: ……………(4) they are at the side of each central incisor

   cuspid: ………………(4) commonly called canine or eye tooth

   bicuspid: ………………(8) the first and second bicuspids

   molars: ………………(8) the first and second molars

   wisdom teeth: ……………(4) the third molars

   A tooth consists of a crown portion, above the gum line, and a root, embedded in the bony tooth socket. The outermost protective layer of the tooth is composed of enamel. Enamel is the hardest substance in the body.

   The heart of each tooth contains living pulp. The pulp contains nerves and blood vessels.

3. **DECIDUOUS TEETH** are primary (baby) teeth.

4. **DENTAL CARIES** are commonly called cavities. They indicate tooth decay.

5. **ABSCESS..OR ABSCESSED TOOTH:** A collection of pus in the pulp of the tooth. The pus displaces and puts pressure on the nerves and blood vessels, causing pain. Treatment usually consists of a root canal. In a root canal, the dentist opens the tooth from above, and cleans the root canal of nerves, blood vessels and debris. The pulp is disinfected and filled with a substance that prevents microorganisms from growing, and the tooth from decaying.

6. **MALOCCLUSION:** In some people the teeth fail to grow in the correct relationship to one another. This can result in incorrect bite, where the teeth make incorrect contact. It can be the cause of many tooth and jaw problems, including TMJ.

7. **TMJ:** is the abbreviation for the temporomandibular joint. The TMJ is a sliding ball and socket joint, located at the point where the lower jaw (the mandible) joins the temporal region of the skull. The joint allows the lower jaw to move. There is a disc in the joint that acts as a shock absorber. The disc provides a gliding action in the joint each time the mouth is opened or closed. Muscles and ligaments help hold the joint in proper alignment.

TOPIC: THE MOUTH AND JAW   (Continued)

8. **TMJ SYNDROME OR DYSFUNCTION:** Pain and other symptoms affecting the head, jaw and face. It is usually the result of years of cumulative problems involving chewing, an incorrect bite, and clenching or grinding the teeth. A severe traumatic injury to the head, neck, or jaw may also precipitate TMJ problems. With the condition of TMJ, the disc no longer glides smoothly. The jaw may click, pop, or grate when the mouth is opened. The jaw may have limited range of motion. X-Rays, MRI and EMG are used for diagnosis. In most cases treatment is aimed at relieving pain and eliminating muscle spasm. Orthodontic work, TMJ splint, and sometimes surgery are treatment options for this condition.

9. **MANDIBLE:** The lower jaw. The most common injury is fracture or dislocation. The mandible joins the temporal bone to form a movable joint.

10. **DISABILITY:** Accidents causing injury to the mouth or jaw can lead to a diagnosis of TMJ. Currently the only rateable finding for TMJ is the injured worker's ability to chew food. The physician will need to specify what type of diet the worker must follow. If the worker is restricted to semi-solid, soft, or liquid foods, impairment is present.

11. **ICD-9:** The most common ICD-9 codes seen in SAIF billings are:

    873.64 ....Tongue laceration

    873.63 ....Broken tooth

    524.6   ....TMJ

    830.0   ....Dislocation, jaw

    802.35 ....Fracture, jaw

Bones of the Skull

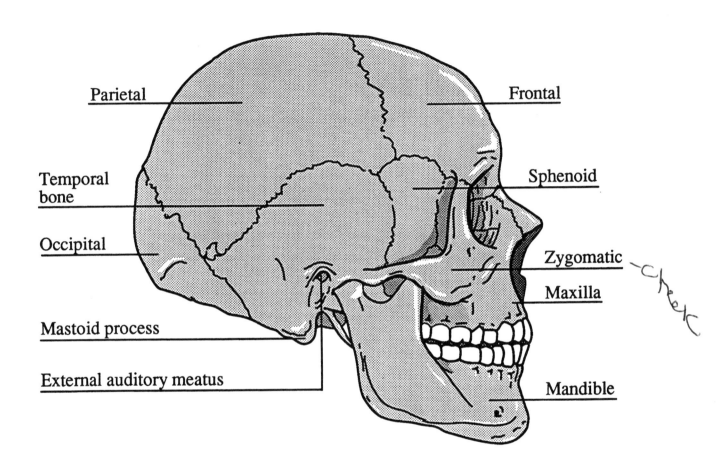

Parietal

Frontal

Temporal
bone

Sphenoid

Occipital

Zygomatic — cheek

Maxilla

Mastoid process

External auditory meatus

Mandible

Skull Base

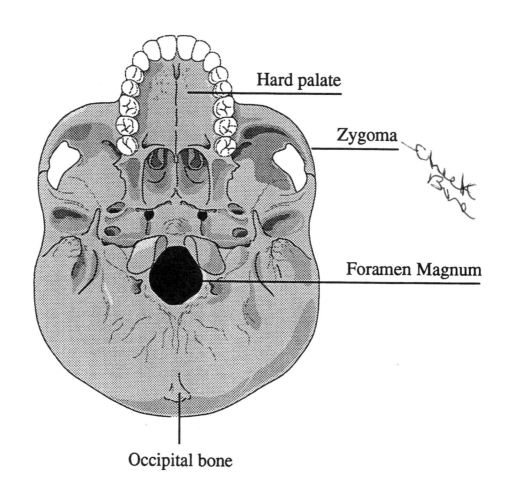

Hard palate

Zygoma

Foramen Magnum

Occipital bone

Sinuses

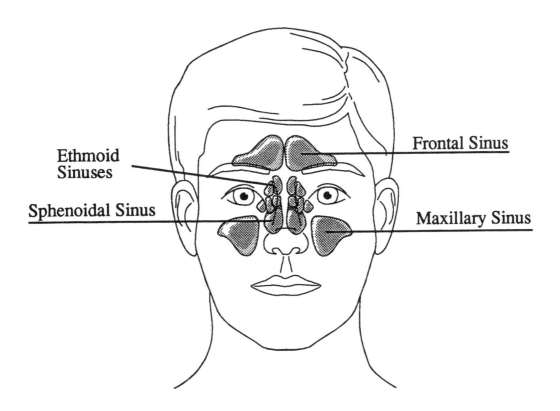

Ethmoid
Sinuses

Sphenoidal Sinus

Frontal Sinus

Maxillary Sinus

Brain

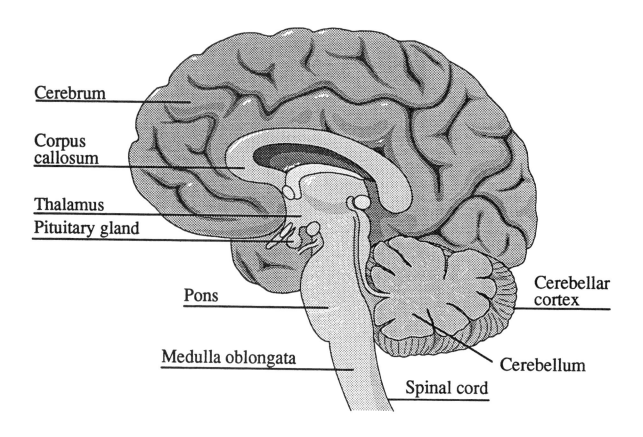

Cerebrum

Corpus
callosum

Thalamus
Pituitary gland

Pons

Medulla oblongata

Cerebellar
cortex

Cerebellum

Spinal cord

Cranial Nerves

I	Olfactory	VII	Facial
II	Optic	VIII	Vestibulocochlear
III	Oculomotor	IX	Glossopharyngeal
IV	Trochlear	X	Vagus
V	Trigeminal	XI	Accessory
VI	Abducens	XII	Hypoglossal

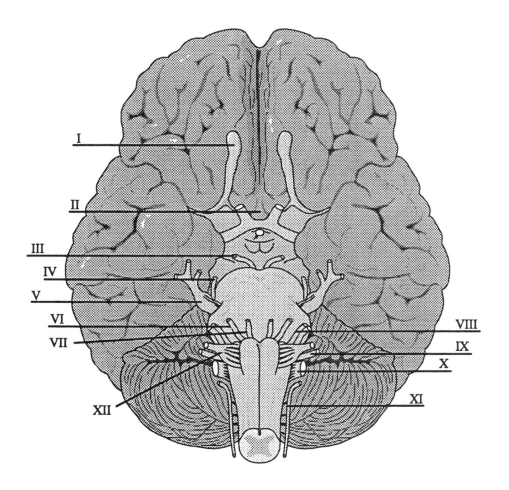

Fig: 1-F

Eye

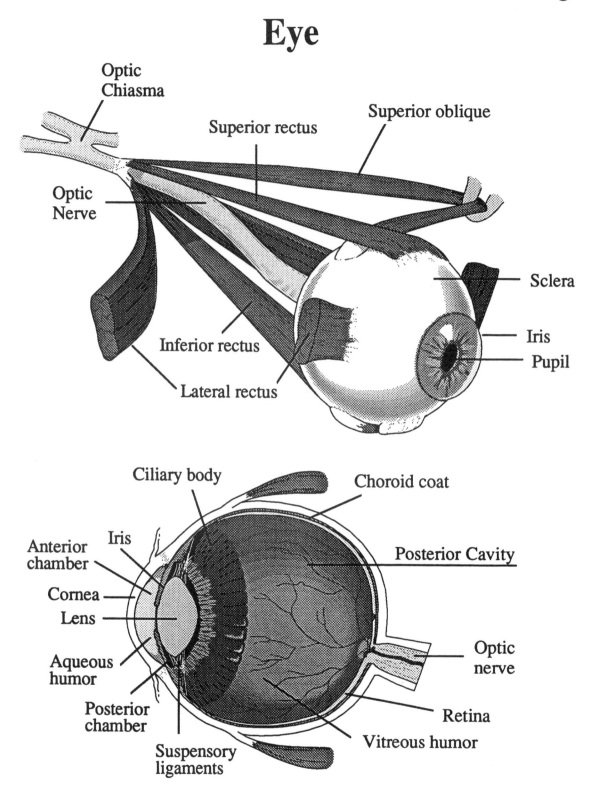

Ear

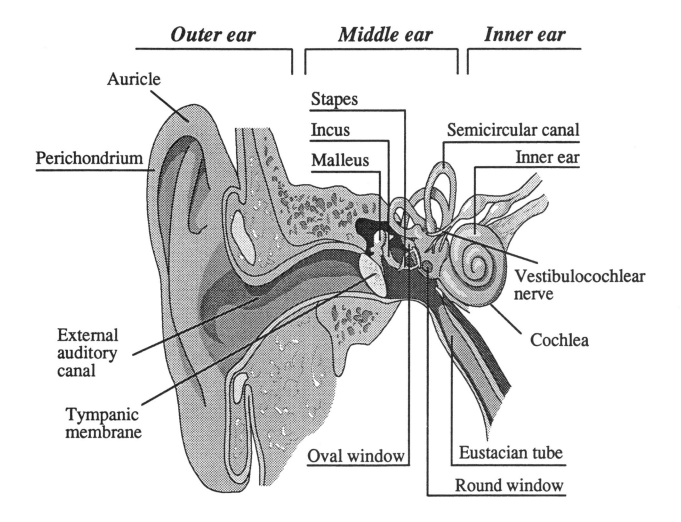

Outer ear | Middle ear | Inner ear

Auricle

Stapes

Incus

Perichondrium

Malleus

Semicircular canal

Inner ear

External
auditory
canal

Vestibulocochlear
nerve

Tympanic
membrane

Cochlea

Oval window

Eustacian tube

Round window

Eustacian Tube and Naso Pharynx

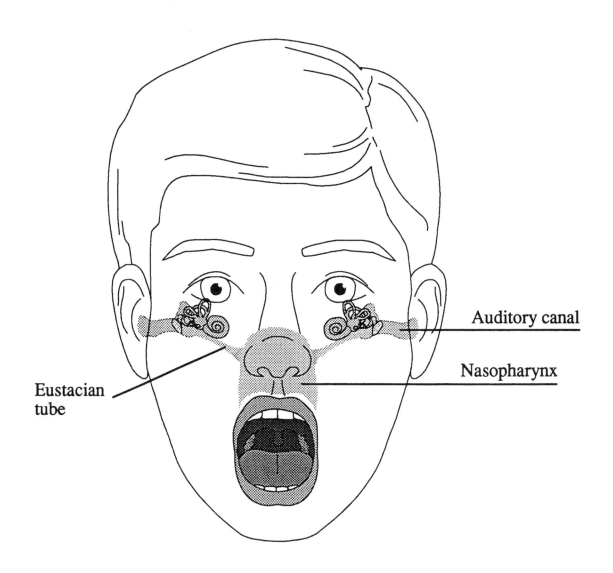

Auditory canal

Nasopharynx

Eustacian
tube

Bones of Skull

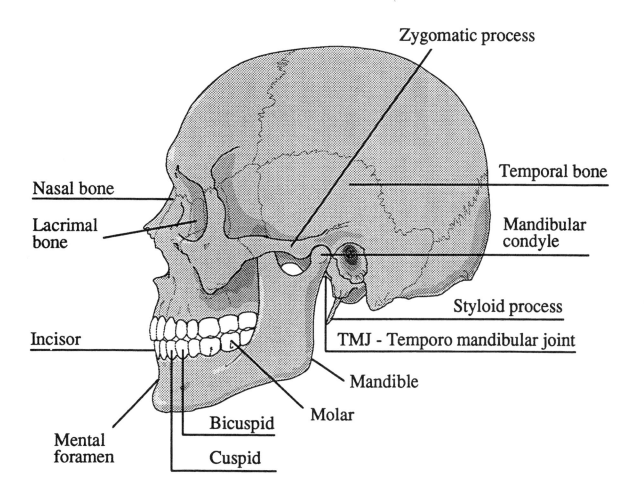

Zygomatic process

Temporal bone

Nasal bone

Lacrimal bone

Mandibular condyle

Styloid process

Incisor

TMJ - Temporo mandibular joint

Mandible

Molar

Bicuspid

Mental foramen

Cuspid

Open Book Quiz:

Name: Kim Dabacon

Session: One

1. Another name for a headache is:

   Cephalgia

2. Name the 3 layers of the meninges. Which is closest to the brain?

   Pia mater - to brain
   Arachnoid - middle
   Dura mater - to skull

3. What is a concussion? An Injury in which the Brain is Violently Shaken.

4. Give 3 immediate symptoms of a concussion.
   - loss of consciousness
   - temporary dizziness
   - disorientation

5. How many pairs of cranial nerves are there?

   12 pairs

6. Name the 10th cranial nerve. Why is it important?

   The Vagus nerve maintains the Rhythmic automatic function of the Internal Body machinery.

7. What is a corneal abrasion?

   A scratch on the cornea.

8. Name two causes of loss of vision.

   Retinal Detachment
   Diabetic Retinopathy

9. What is conductive hearing impairment?

   a problem in the external or middle ear.

10. Give 3 symptoms of TMJ syndrome. What does TMJ stand for? Temporomandibular joint.
    1. Incorrect Bite
    2. clenching
    3. grinding the teeth

11. Describe a depressed basal skull fracture.
    a piece of Bone is driven inward and presses on the Brain

12. Describe a epidural hematoma. Is it serious? — yes, —
    a Blood clot on or above the Dura Mater.

13. Can an injury cause glaucoma?
    — yes, a trauma.

Medical Basics

TOPIC: SKIN...Dermatology   (Derm...root word for skin)
                                     (Cutis...root word for skin)

1. **The skin is the largest body organ.** The average adult has over 3000 square inches of skin surface. It weighs about six pounds. 1/3 of all the blood circulating through the body is circulating through the skin.

2. **Functions:**

    – Protects deeper tissues against drying and invasion by organisms

    – Protects more sensitive tissues in the body against injury

    – Regulates body temperature

    – Protects against loss of moisture

    – It's nerve endings continually obtain and relay information about the environment

3. **Structure:**
    3 layers...epidermis, dermis, subcutaneous tissue

    Located in those layers are:

    – Sensory cells that keep the brain and other organs aware of the environment

    – Nerve endings that register pain and pleasure

    – Sweat glands

    – Sebaceous glands

    – Hairs

    – Arterioles and venules

4. **Accessory organs of the skin are the hair, nails and glands.**
    Hair is a thread like structure composed of dead cells. The cells are filled with a tough, protein substance called keratin. A substance called melanin in the hair shaft is responsible for hair color.

    Nails are composed of hard, curved plates of keratin.

    Glands, such as sebaceous and sweat, manufacture and discharge a secretion.

5. **Sweat..Why do people sweat?**
    The human body has a built in thermostat. Sweating is part of the system that keeps the body cool. Here's how the system works...tiny openings in the skin called sweat glands are located all over the body. The palms and soles of the feet have the highest concentration of sweat glands. These glands loop and coil deep in the skin. Some of the fluid from around the blood vessels is drawn off and passed into the sweat glands, and then out to the skin. Cooling results when the sweat evaporates from the surface of the skin.

TOPIC: SKIN…Dermatology (Continued)

6. **Types of abnormality of the skin surface..these are called skin lesions:**

   macule ……………….flat, discolored spot (freckles, measles, tattoos)

   papule ………………solid, elevated lesion (wart, moles)

   nodule ………………a solid lesion that may or may not be elevated (cyst, lipoma)

   vesicle ………………a round, elevated lesion containing serous fluid (mosquito bite)

   pustule ………………same, but contains pus (acne, carbuncles)

   keloid ………………scar

7. **Dermatitis: inflammation of the skin.** Dermatitis can be caused by anything that causes the skin to be irritated or inflamed. The main types of dermatitis are:

   Seborrheic …………the most common variety is dandruff, but it can also form a red scaly rash on the face, back or chest. May be related to stress.

   Contact dermatitis …Contact dermatitis is a response of the skin as a result of local contact with one or more irritating, allergic, or photosensitizing chemical agents. Prime causes in the workplace are chemicals, detergents, plants.

   Latex gloves.

   Eczema ……………inflammation of the skin, usually accompanied by scaling or blisters. It is sometimes caused by an allergy, but may also occur for no known reason.

8. **Fungal infection of the skin is common.** Treatment is rarely related to a work injury:

   Tinea ………………also called ringworm. Physicians often follow the diagnosis of tinea, with the Latin word for the location..as in:

   Tinea pedis (feet) …Tinea pedis is also called athlete's foot.

   Tinea cruris…………jock itch

   Tinea unguium. ……ringworm of the fingernails or toenails, also called onychomycosis (on-y-cho-my-cosis).

9. **ICD-9 codes commonly:**

   692.0 ………………dermatitis due to detergents

   692.1…………………dermatitis due to oil and grease

   692.6…………………dermatitis due to plants

   686.9…………………local skin infection

Itching of the skin is — PRURITIS
Infection of the skin — is — Cellulitis

TOPIC: BURNS

1. **In the United States each year, there are approximately 70,000 people burned badly enough to require hospitalization. These burns are most commonly from fire, chemicals, and electricity.**

2. **The skin is living tissue;** even a brief exposure to temperatures of 120 degrees can damage the cells in the three layers: epidermis, dermis and subcutaneous tissue.

3. **First-degree (superficial burn)** effects only the outer layer.

   > Produces a red discoloration of the skin, as in a sunburn
   >
   > Usually heals quickly, with no scarring.
   >
   > A friction burn is an example. ICD-9: 913.1 (forearm or wrist).
   >
   > Symptoms may include headache, pain and fever.

   Second-degree (partial thickness burn) effects some of the dermis, but some of the dermis is left to recover. It will produce blisters, and severe pain if burn is close to the surface of the skin. It produces loss of sensation if the burn is deeper. (blisters occur when fluid is lost from blood vessels, and becomes trapped beneath the skin.)

   It usually heals in five to thirty days, and can heal without scarring. If 10 percent of the body is burned, medical treatment is necessary, or shock may prove fatal.

   Third-degree burn (full thickness burn) destroys the full skin thickness.
   It will produce white, leathery, charred, dry skin. If deep enough, the bones and muscles may be exposed. It will destroy hair follicles, blood vessels, and nerve endings. The tissue may coagulate, with little or no pain. There is slow healing, with scarring. Skin grafts may be needed.

   If 10 percent of the body is burned, medical treatment is necessary, or shock may prove fatal.

4. **Complications:** In second or third degree burns, the injured person will be in shock if more than 10 percent of the body surface is affected. The shock will produce low blood pressure. This is brought on by the loss of large amounts of fluid from the burned area. If this fluid is not replaced by IV's, it may be fatal.

5. **Burned skin can no longer protect the body from infective organisms.**
   Effective antibiotic treatment is necessary to combat the fatal effects of infection.

   Victims who have inhaled smoke may have complications involving their lungs.
   Eyes may also have problems. ICD-9: 940.0 chemical burns of the eye.

6. **Electrical burns may have extensive internal damage, with little external damage.**
   They require examination by a physician, as heart damage may result.
   ICD-9: 944.00 - electric shock burn of the hand.

TOPIC: NECK

1. The back (posterior portion) of the neck contains the bony structure of the cervical vertebrae, which encloses the upper portion of the spinal cord. The front (anterior portion) of the neck contains the pharynx, larynx, esophagus, and trachea. Large arteries and veins are located on either side of the neck. The thyroid gland is located at the base of the neck.

> **Pharynx** ....Connects the back of the mouth to the esophagus. Swallowed food travels down the pharynx.
>
> **Larynx**.................The voice box. It is responsible for voice production and keeps swallowed food from entering the airway.
>
> **Esophagus** ....A muscular tube leading from mouth to the stomach.

2. **Functions of the neck include:**

    - Supporting and facilitating movement of the head.

    - It's an avenue for the blood supply to the brain.

    - It houses the airway and food pathway.

3. **Whiplash is a common injury to the neck.** It's caused by a sudden forceful thrust of the head backward (hyperextension), forward (hyperflexion), and sometimes sideways. Muscle and ligament damage may result. Severe whiplash may jar the brain, producing minute hemorrhages on it's surface. Severe injury may also result in spinal cord injury, or even death. Whiplash is a frequent injury that may occur to a person in a vehicle that is suddenly, forcibly struck from the rear.

4. **Blood supply:** The carotid arteries and the jugular veins are found in the neck.

TOPIC: BONES   (OSTEO = Root word for bone)

1. **Bones provide a rigid framework for the body.** They contain calcium and phosphorus to make them hard and rigid. All bones are structured in the same way:

   The surface is covered with a thin membrane called periosteum.

   Then comes a hard, dense shell of bone material.

   Inside that shell is a spongy material.

   The spongy material surrounds the bone marrow.

2. **Bone marrow:** Soft, fatty tissue found in bone cavities. Bone marrow produces blood cells. It produces all the red blood cells, platelets, and most of the white blood cells.

3. **Bone is insensitive.** Sensations arise from the nerves in the periosteum.

4. **Processes on bone:**

   Bone head ....Rounded end of a bone.

   Tubercle ....Small rounded area for attachment of tendons or muscles.

   Tuberosity ....Large, rounded area for attachment of tendons or muscles.

   Condyle ....Knuckle-like process at the joint.

5. **Depressions in bone:**

   Fossa ....Depression or cavity in a bone.

   Foramen ....Opening for blood vessels and nerves.

   Fissure ....A narrow, deep slit-like opening.

   Sulcus ....A groove or furrow.

   Sinus ....Cavity within a bone.

TOPIC: JOINTS   (ARTH, ARTHR, ARTHRO = Root word for joint)

1. **A joint is formed at the point where two bones meet.** Some joints are fixed, as are those suture lines in the skull. Some joints allow limited movement, as with the vertebrae. Highly mobile joints are responsible for body movement. Three types of highly mobile joints are:

    Hinge joints............located in the elbows and knees.

    Ball-and-socket ......located in the shoulder and hip.

    Pivot joint ....allows rotation, as in turning the head side to side.

2. **Freely movable joints are also called synovial joints.** The surface of the bones at these joints is covered with smooth cartilage. The bones are separated by a joint capsule. Ligaments anchor the bones together around the joint capsule. Synovial membrane lines the capsule of the joint, and secretes a lubricating fluid called synovial fluid, which reduces the friction of movement.

3. **Joints can develop many problems.** Some of the most common are:

    Arthritis ....Inflammation of a joint.

    Dislocation ....Complete displacement of 2 bones.
    It is usually accompanied by tearing of the joints ligaments.

    Subluxation............A partial dislocation of a joint.

4. **Bursitis is the inflammation of a bursa.** It may occur following a strain or irritation. The bursa is a small fluid filled sac that acts as a cushion where a tendon or muscle crosses a bone or other muscle. The most important bursas are around the shoulder, elbow and knee joints. A bursa is lined with synovial membrane, and is filled with synovial fluid.

5. **Joints will be discussed more thoroughly in the sections on the back and knee.**

TOPIC: TERMS OF MOVEMENT

1. **Flexion** ....The act of bending

2. **Extension** ....The act of straightening

3. **Adduction** ....Bringing a part of the body toward the midline of the body

4. **Abduction** ....Moving away from the midline of the body

5. **Rotation** ....The act of turning on an axis (as in turning the head)

6. **Elevation** ....The act of raising a part

7. **Depression** ....The lowering of a part

TOPIC: TERMS OF DIRECTION

1. **Anterior** ....Toward the front

2. **Posterior** ....Toward the back

3. **Lateral** ....To the side

4. **Medial** ....To the middle

5. **Proximal** ....Nearest the body trunk

6. **Distal** ....Far from the body trunk, or distant part of a limb

7. **Superior** ....Upward

8. **Inferior** ....Downward

9. **Oblique** ....Slanting

10. **Prone** ....Face downward

11. **Supine** ....Face upward

Medical Basics — Chapter 2

TOPIC: BONES OF UPPER TRUNK

1. **Bones of the upper trunk include:** Clavicle or collar bone (2), Sternum or breast bone (1), Scapula or shoulder blade (2), Ribs (12 pair), Vertebrae (12 in the thoracic spine).

2. **Clavicle:** Extends from the breast bone to the arm, also called the collar bone.

3. **Scapula:** Joins the clavicle. It is a large, triangular bone, also called the shoulder blade.

4. **Sternum:** Known as the breast bone. It's a long, narrow, somewhat flat bone that forms the center front of the chest.

5. **Ribs:** There are 12 pair of ribs. They all extend from the vertebra in the thoracic spine around to various positions in the front of the chest. They form the rib cage, or as it's sometimes called, the thorax. There are 12 pair:

    7 pair join the sternum in front, (called true ribs).

    3 pair do not attach to the sternum, (called false ribs).

    2 bottom pair are called floating ribs.

    The first 7 pair of ribs are connected to the sternum by costal cartilage. The costal cartilage are flexible and allow for chest expansion when breathing.

    Ribs protect the organs in the chest. A fractured rib can be painful. It can cause damage if the sharp pieces of bone puncture underlying structures, such as the spleen or lung.

6. **Common ICD-9 codes:**

    875.0....................Open wound of chest wall

    922.1....................Contusion of chest wall*

7. **Contusion:** A bruise. The skin is not broken with this type of injury.

TOPIC: UPPER EXTREMITIES

1. **The humerus is the long bone in the upper arm.** Anatomically speaking, the "arm" is what we refer to as the upper arm.

2. **The lower arm is called the forearm.** It contains 2 bones: The radius and ulna. The radius is found on the same side as the thumb.

3. **Bones of the hand are divided into three areas:**

   Carpals ....Wrist bones

   Metacarpals ....The body of the hand

   Phalanges ....The fingers. Individual bones are called a phalanx. The phalanx are called proximal, middle, and distal.

4. **The elbow is the joint between the lower end of the humerus and the upper ends of the radius and ulna.** It is stabilized by ligaments at the front and back.

   The olecranon is a bony projection forming the point of the elbow. It's commonly called the "funny bone". Olecranon bursitis can occur in response to local irritation.

5. **The shoulder is formed at the juncture of the scapula, clavicle, and humerus.**

6. **The acromioclavicular joint is formed where the clavicle meets the acromion on the scapula.** The acromion is a bony prominence on the upper, shoulder side of the scapula.

7. **Just below the acromion, on the outer wall of the scapula, is the glenoid cavity.** The head of the humerus fits into the glenoid cavity to form the shoulder joint.

8. **The shoulder joint is a ball and socket joint.**

9. **The rotator cuff is a reinforcing structure around the shoulder joint composed of four muscle tendons that merge with the fibrous capsule enclosing the joint.** Degenerative changes of age and use can cause a thinning of the rotator cuff, making it more susceptible to injury. Overhead work or sudden shoulder exertion are common causes of rotator cuff injury, sometimes causing it to tear. Injury to the rotator cuff may require surgical repair. An arthrogram or an MRI are useful in diagnosing a rotator cuff tear. These diagnostic studies will also identify edema of the rotator cuff.

10. **The Carpal Tunnel is a space within the palm side of the hand and wrist.** Passing through this space are 9 flexor tendons and the median nerve. Carpal tunnel syndrome is a fairly common diagnosis. It can indicate cumulative trauma, or overuse syndrome. Other causes, or contributing factors, can include obesity, diabetes, pregnancy, arthritis, or fractures. It's symptoms include numbness and tingling along the median nerve root distribution. Tinel's and Phalen's sign, Electromyogram (EMG), and nerve conduction studies (NCS), provide objective evidence of nerve compromise.

TOPIC: UPPER EXTREMITIES (Continued)

11. Nerves of the upper extremity:

Brachial Plexus ......A network of lower cervical and upper thoracic spinal nerves supplying the arm, forearm and hand.

Median nerve ....Originates in the brachial plexus. It innervates the forearm.

Ulnar nerve ....Innervates the muscles and skin of forearm and hand.

Radial Nerve ....Innervates the skin of the back of the entire arm and hand.

12. Blood Supply:

Radial artery ....Pulse at the wrist. It supplies the forearm, wrist, hand.

Brachial artery ......Pulse at the elbow. It supplies the upper arm.

13. Muscles:

Biceps ....Flexes upper arm.

Deltoid ....Raises and rotates arm.

Triceps.................Extends arm and forearm.

14. Diagnostic tests:

Biceps Reflex ....Front elbow reflex. Used to test the C5 nerve root.

Tinel's ....Tests ulnar, radial, or median nerves for injury or pathology. A positive Tinel's indicates that further diagnostic studies are necessary.

Phalen's ....Indicates carpal tunnel compression syndrome if numbness and tingling of the fingers is produced. A positive Phalen's may indicate that further diagnostic studies are necessary.

15. Definitions:

Tendon.................Fibrous connective tissue attaching muscle to bone. It is very strong, and will not stretch.

Ligament ....fibrous connective tissue attaching bone to bone. The fibers will stretch.

Strain ....A muscle tear. It is graded according to severity:

Grade I: Stretching a few muscle fibers, with minimal tearing.

Grade II: Partial tear of muscle fibers, creating a muscle defect that can be felt on exam.

Grade III: Extensive tear or complete rupture.

TOPIC: UPPER EXTREMITIES (Continued)

Sprain ....A ligament tear. It usually involves a joint, and requires longer healing time than a strain. Is graded according to severity (I, II, III).

Origin/insertion ......When muscles join bones, one of the bones usually serves as an anchor to help move the other bone. The point where the muscle joins the anchor bone is called the origin. Where it attaches to the bone that moves, it's called the insertion. The origin of the biceps is on the shoulder, and the insertion is on the radius, just below the elbow. The origin of the triceps is at the shoulder also, but it runs behind the elbow, and has it's insertion in the ulna.

Tendon sheaths ......The sheaths are tunnels that keep tendons close to the bones they move. They also protect the tendons.

16. Common ICD-9 codes:

354.0....................Carpal tunnel.

883.0....................Open wound, finger.

927.20 ....Crush injury, hand.

353.0....................Brachial plexus lesion (lesion = injury or wound).

17. Disability:

Shoulder ....Rotator cuff tear is quite common. Surgery is rateable for removal of any of the acromion or the distal clavicle. Weakness on the affected side is a standard finding at closure.

Carpal tunnel ....CT surgery is not rateable. However, loss of strength is. Many files are now being closed with PPD for strength loss. This is due to physicians becoming more aware that this should be demonstrated on closing reports.

"Other findings"......Sensory loss, arm length discrepancies, surgeries, strength, dermatological problems, and vascular problems need to be addressed in closing reports.

TOPIC: COMMON DISORDERS OF THE UPPER EXTREMITIES

1. **CUMULATIVE TRAUMA DISORDER** is a term used to identify the group of musculoskeletal disorders involving injuries to the tendons, tendon sheaths, and related bones. Repetitive movement and cumulative work stress imposed on these movements can result in disorders such as tendinitis, tenosynovitis, epicondylitis, and carpal tunnel syndrome.
These are all examples of cumulative trauma disorders.

2. **TENOSYNOVITIS** is the inflammation of the tendons and their sheaths. It commonly occurs at the wrist.

3. **DEQUERVAINS DISEASE** can occur when the tendon sheath of both the long and short abductor muscles of the thumb narrows at the wrist junction. Tenosynovitis of this area creates pain in the side of the thumb and side of the wrist.

4. **TRIGGER FINGER.** Tenosynovitis causes a finger or thumb to have problems flexing or extending. Movement is temporarily arrested, but then completes the motion with a jerk.

5. **TENDONITIS** is inflammation of a tendon. It remains one of the more common joint diseases.

6. **EPICONDYLITIS (TENNIS ELBOW)** is a form of tendonitis to the tissues in the elbow. It is caused by excessive strain to the muscles of the forearm which attach at the elbow. Pain is located at the elbow and extends down the forearm.

7. **CARPAL TUNNEL SYNDROME** is caused by compression of the median nerve in the carpal tunnel. The carpal tunnel is a small area in the wrist that must accommodate the finger flexor tendons and the median nerve as they pass from the forearm into the hand. Injury results in impaired or lost nerve function in the first 3 1/2 fingers and part of the thumb.

   Facts:

   It occurs more frequently in women than men (ratio: 5-1).

   Symptoms include numbness (night numbness in particular), tingling, pain in the hand.

   There may also be weakness in the muscles of the thumb.

   Surgery may be necessary if conservative treatment fails.

8. **GANGLION.** A cystic swelling overlying a joint or tendon sheath. It is found most frequently at the wrist. A cyst is a closed sac or pouch, with a definite wall, that contains some fluid, that may become solid. It may appear gradually or suddenly. It disappear, only to come back again. When the cyst is connected with the tendon sheath, the affected finger may feel weak. The dorsum of the wrist is the most common location.

TOPIC: COMMON DISORDERS OF THE UPPER EXTREMITIES
(Continued)

9. **NEUROMA.** Is a tumor composed of nerve cells. It can form at the end of a severed nerve.

10. **COLLES' FRACTURE.** A break in the radius, just above the wrist.
    It is the most common fracture in people over 40.
    It usually results when a person falls forward with their arm outstretched.

11. **ADHESIVE CAPSULITIS** is an inflammation of the shoulder joint capsule and the peripheral articular cartilage. Symptoms include decreased range of motion (ROM), swelling over the AC joint, and pain with joint movement.

Skin

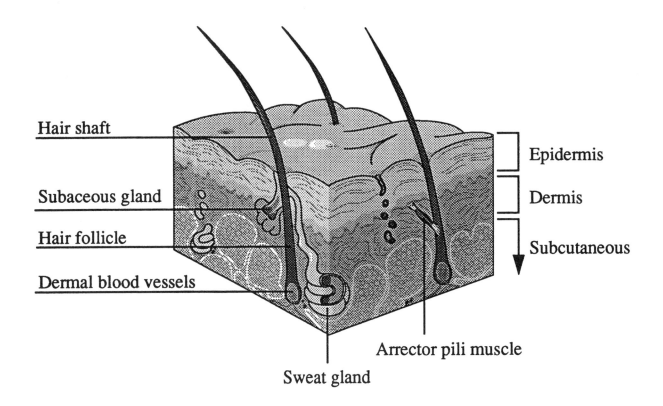

Hair shaft

Subaceous gland

Hair follicle

Dermal blood vessels

Epidermis

Dermis

Subcutaneous

Sweat gland

Arrector pili muscle

Ribs

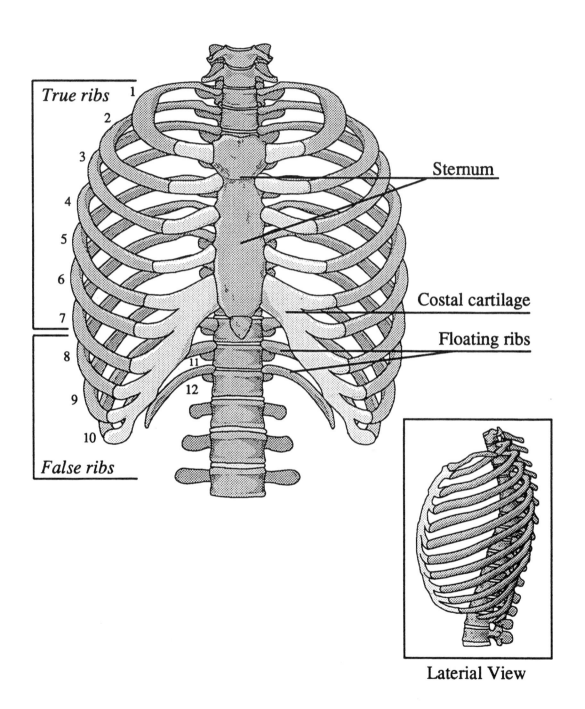

True ribs 1
2
3
4
5
6
7

Sternum

Costal cartilage

Floating ribs

False ribs
8
9
10
11
12

Laterial View

Joints of the Upper Extremity

Shoulder

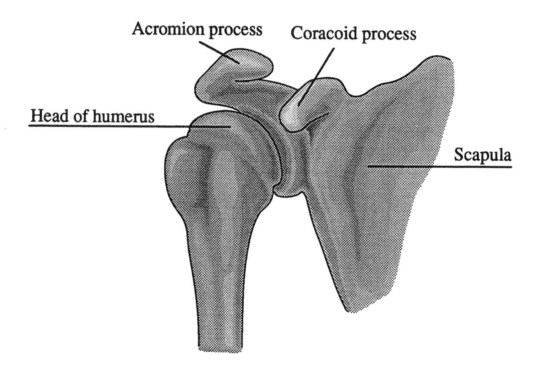

Acromion process

Coracoid process

Head of humerus

Scapula

Anterior Arm

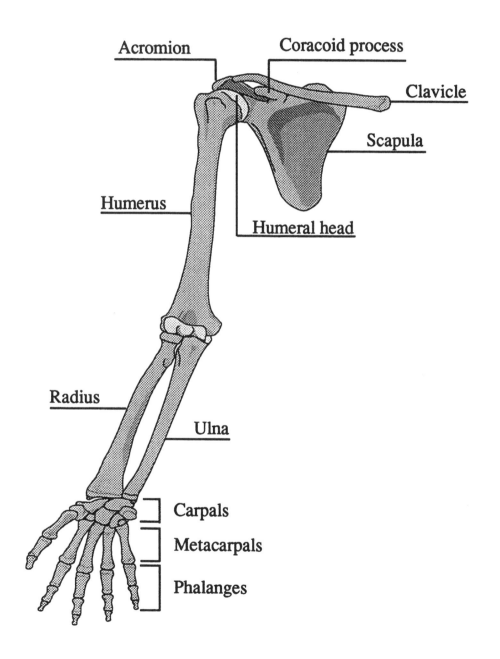

Acromion   Coracoid process

Clavicle

Scapula

Humerus

Humeral head

Radius

Ulna

Carpals

Metacarpals

Phalanges

Joints of the Upper Extremity

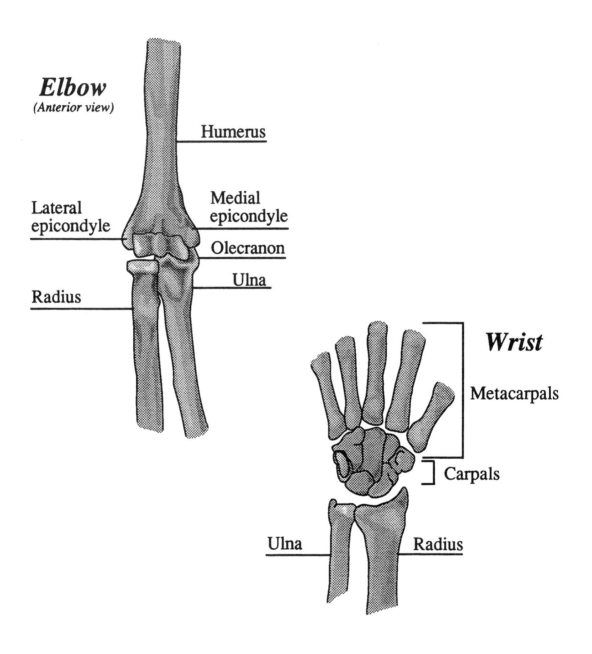

Elbow
(Anterior view)

Humerus

Lateral
epicondyle

Medial
epicondyle

Olecranon

Ulna

Radius

Wrist

Metacarpals

Carpals

Ulna

Radius

Hand

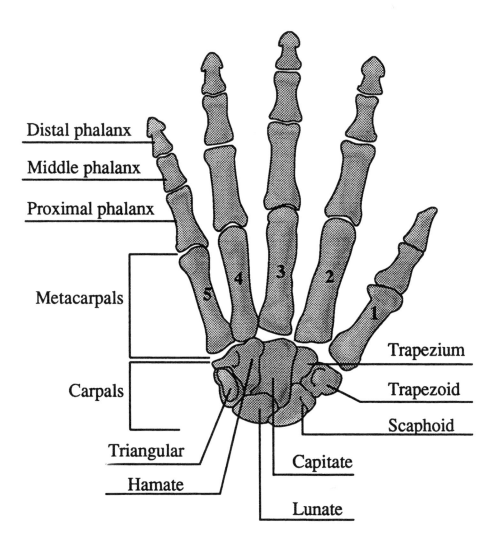

Distal phalanx

Middle phalanx

Proximal phalanx

Metacarpals

Carpals

Triangular

Hamate

Trapezium

Trapezoid

Scaphoid

Capitate

Lunate

Medical Basics

Chapter 2

Open Book Quiz:

Name: Kim Dabacon

Session: 2

1. Name the three layers of skin:
   - epidermis
   - dermis
   - subcutaneous tissue

2. What is whiplash?

   a common injury to the neck.

3. Name two types of joints, and give an example of where each is located in the body.
   - Hidge Joints - in the Elbows + knees
   - Ball & Socket Joints - in the shoulder + hip

4. Define the words medial and distal.
   - medial - to the middle
   - distal - far from the body trunk, or distant part of a limb.

5. How does a second degree burn differ from a third degree burn?
   - Second degree is a partial thickness burn.
   - third degree is a full thickness of the skin burn.

6. What three bones form the shoulder?
   - Scapula
   - Clavicle
   - humerus

7. What is a rotator cuff tear? How is it diagnosed?

   a tear is a result from overhead work or sudden exertion.
   It's diagnosed by an arthrogram or MRI.

8. Where is the carpal tunnel? What nerve goes through it?
   - a space in the palm side of the hand + wrist

   - The median nerve.

9. What is the difference between a sprain and a strain?
   - Sprain - is a ligament tear
   - Strain - is a muscle tear

10. What is the difference between a tendon and a ligament?

    Tendon attachs muscle to bone is very strong + will not stretch.

    Ligament attachs bone to bone + the fibers stretch.

50

Medical Basics

TOPIC: THE PELVIS

1. **The pelvis is formed by the sacrum, coccyx, and the pelvic girdle.**

2. **The pelvic girdle consists of 2 bones, commonly known as hip bones.**

3. **Each hip bone is composed of bones called the ilium, ischium, and pubis.** These parts fuse together in the region of a cup-shaped cavity called the acetabulum. The acetabulum is located on the lateral surface of the hip bone, and is part of the joint that receives the rounded end of the femur.

4. **The ilium is the uppermost portion of the hipbone.** The uppermost prominence of the ilium is the iliac crest. Posteriorly, the ilium joins the sacrum at the sacroiliac joint. This is sometimes referred to as the SI joint.

5. **The ischium forms the lowest portion of the hip bone.**

6. **The front portion of the coxal bone is the pubis.** The two pubic bones come together at the midline to create a joint called the symphysis pubis.

7. **The sacrum and coccyx are pelvic bones that are also part of the spine.** The sacrum is at the back of the pelvis, and is shaped like an inverted triangle. The coccyx is at the distal tip of the sacrum, and is called the tailbone.

8. **Function:** The pelvis provides support for the trunk of the body and attachments for the legs. It protects the bladder, the distal end of the large intestine, and the internal reproductive organs.

TOPIC: URINARY SYSTEM

1. **The urinary system includes the kidneys, ureters, urinary bladder, and urethra.**

2. **The kidneys are located retroperitoneally** (behind the peritoneal membrane that lines the wall of the abdominal cavity), against the deep muscles of the back. The primary function of the kidney is to remove waste from the circulatory system. Other functions include:

   Assists in control of the rate of red blood cell formation.

   Helps regulate blood pressure by secreting renin.

   Regulates the absorption of calcium.

3. **Ureters carry urine from the kidney to the bladder.**

4. **Composition of urine: 95% water, body wastes, urea and creatinine.**

5. **Micturition and voiding are two medical words that describe the process of urine leaving the body.**

6. **Various problems in the urinary tract may result in a symptom of low back pain.**
   These could include infection or renal calculi (kidney stone).

7. **Vocabulary:**

   Urologist ....MD specializing in treatment of the urinary tract.

   Cystitis...................................Inflammation of the urinary bladder

   Diuretic..................................A substance that causes an increased production of urine.

   Hematuria ....Blood in the urine.

   Incontinence.........................Inability to control the urination/defecation reflex

   Nephrectomy.........................Surgical removal of a kidney.

   U.T.I. ....Urinary tract infection

8. **Common ICD-9 codes:**

   866.00.................................Kidney Injury

   599.0....................................Urinary Tract Infection (UTI)

TOPIC: STRUCTURES PROTECTED BY THE BONY FRAMEWORK OF THE PELVIS

Distal End of the Large Intestine

1. **The distal end of the large intestine composes the lower portion of the alimentary canal.** The individual structures are: the cecum, the colon, rectum, and anal canal.

2. **It's primary function is the transportation of the residues of food digestion from the digestive process to elimination.** The residue is called stool or feces. The process of elimination is called defecation.

Internal Reproductive Organs

Both male and female reproductive organs are located in the pelvis.

Basic structural differences exist between the male and female pelvis. The differences are related to the function of the pelvis as a birth canal. In the female, the iliac bones are more flared creating more internal area. The female pelvis is usually lighter, more fragile, and shows less evidence of muscle attachments than the male pelvis.

Complaints of back pain can result from problems with the internal structures in both men and women. (Pain felt in one area, when it originates in another area, is called referred pain.)

ICD-9 codes most commonly seen for the lower trunk:

922.2............................Contusion, Abdominal wall

942.03........................Burn, Abdominal wall

TOPIC: HERNIA

1. **A hernia occurs when all or part of an organ protrudes through the wall of the cavity in which it's usually contained.**

2. **Hernias most commonly occur in the lower abdomen, when some part of intestine protrudes outside it's normal boundary. 80 percent of all hernias are inguinal hernias.**

3. **In most cases, the hernia develops from a natural defect in physical development.** This happens in approximately 1/4 of the male population when the inguinal canal does not seal itself completely after the testes have descended into the scrotum. A hernia in this area is called an inguinal hernia.

4. **Indirect inguinal hernia:** Occurs when a loop of intestine is forced into the inguinal canal. The intestine can sometimes descend into the scrotum.

5. **Direct inguinal hernia**: Occurs when the intestine protrudes through the intestinal wall.

6. **Femoral hernial:** A loop of intestine slips into the femoral ring. The femoral ring is an area that allows the large blood vessels and nerves to pass from the trunk to the lower extremity.

7. **Strangulated hernia:** Occurs if the protruding intestinal loop is so tightly constricted that the blood supply is interrupted. Without prompt treatment, the strangulated tissues may die.

8. **Hernias usually develop gradually.** Because of this they are relatively painless. Often, they are totally asymptomatic and unknown to the individual until a bulge becomes apparent. Hernias do not normally result from a single incident. They may, however, be discovered as the result of a single incident.

9. **Hernias have often been blamed on "lifting something too heavy".** Many times the hernia was present, but unknown and totally asymptomatic, until the bulge became apparent.

10. **A Hiatal hernia** is present when a portion of the stomach protrudes upward through a weaked area in musculature of the diaphragm.

11. **Common ICD-9 Codes:**

    550.90.........................Inguinal hernia

    553.00.........................Femoral hernia

TOPIC: LOWER EXTREMITIES

1. **Bones of the Leg, ankle, instep and toes:**

   Femur (1): .... The thigh bone, femur, is the longest, strongest bone in the body.

   Patella (1): ....The knee-cap, a flat bone on the anterior surface of the knee.

   Tibia (1): ....One of two bones in the lower leg. Located on the medial side, between knee and ankle.

   Fibula (1): ....The other bone in the lower leg. Located on the lateral side, between knee and ankle.

   Tarsal (7): ....Ankle

   Metatarsal (5): ....Instep

   Phalanx (14): ....Toe

2. **The head of the femur fits into the pelvis in a cavity called the acetabulum.** Through the acetabulum, the femur bears the weight of the body. The acetabulum also plays a significant role in our ability to walk.

3. At the lower end of the femur, two rounded processes, **the lateral and medial condyles**, articulate with the tibia of the lower leg.

4. The patella articulates with the femur on its distal anterior surface.

5. The **tibia**, or shinbone, is the larger of the two lower leg bones and is located on the medial side. At the distal end, the tibia expands to form a prominence on the inner ankle called the **medial malleolus**.

6. The **fibula** is a long, slender bone located on the lateral side of the tibia. The fibula does not enter into the knee joint and does not bear any body weight.

7. The **foot** consists of the **ankle, instep, and five toes.**

   The ankle's seven bones form a group called the tarsus. The bones areso arranged, that one of them, the talus, can move freely where it joins the tibia and fibula. The largest of the anklebones, the calcaneus, or heel bone, is just below the talus, forming the base of the heel.

   The instep consists of five elongated metatarsal bones

   The phalanges of the toes are similar to those of the fingers.

TOPIC: LOWER EXTREMITIES (Continued)

8. **Fractures commonly occur at the femoral head, neck, and acetabulum.**
   A fracture in any of these places is called a hip fracture. The incidence of hip fractures increases with age. These fractures can require a lengthy recovery period.

9. **The femur is the most important weight-bearing bone in the body.** When fractured, it's size makes healing difficult. The blood vessels to the femur are small in relation to the area of bone they supply. Most femoral fractures are oblique. Healing is sometimes prolonged because the weight of the femur tends to pull the bone fragments apart.

10. **A healed fracture is called a bony union.**

11. **Most fractures of the femur will be repaired by open reduction (surgery).** The surgery can include the use of metal plates or pins to aid in holding the fractured bone together and speed up the healing time.

12. **The femur attaches to the hip at the acetablum.**
    This ball and socket joint form one of the largest weight bearing joints in the body. In a healthy hip, smooth cartilage covers the ends of these bones, allowing for smooth, painless movement. If that cartilage "cushion" wears away, and the bones rub together, the bone becomes roughened. This   creates pain and stiffness. Surgical treatment is sometimes done to replace the worn out socket. The procedure is called a total hip replacement. The prosthesis will allow a person to move easily without pain. ROM (range of motion) may be limited following this type of surgical replacement.

13. **Common ICD-9 Codes:**

   820.00..........................Fractured Femur

   682.6............................Cellulitis of the Leg*
                             *(Cellulitis = inflammation spreads beyond a localized area.)

   897.4............................Amputated leg

TOPIC: KNEE

1. **The knee-joint is formed where the femur and tibia come together (articulate).**
   It is covered anteriorly with the patella or kneecap. The articulating surfaces of the femur and tibia are separated by the two menisci (sometimes called semilunar cartilage). There are also several bursae associated with the knee joint.

2. **The knee is the largest and most complex of the synovial joints.**
   Here is the general structure of a synovial joint:

   A. Articular ends of the bones are covered with a thin layer of cartilage. The cartilage is resistant to wear, and produces minimal friction when the joint is moved.

   B. The bones are held together by a joint capsule. This is composed of dense, white, fibrous tissue that attaches to the periosteum of the bones near the articular end. The capsule completely encases the other parts of the joint.

   C. Ligaments reinforce the capsule, and help bind the bones together. These include the anterior and posterior cruciate, the lateral and medial collateral, and the patellar ligament.

   D. On the inside of the joint, there's a shiny vascular lining of loose connective tissue called the synovial membrane. This membrane surrounds a closed sac, called the synovial cavity. Into this cavity, the joint secretes synovial fluid.

   E. Synovial fluid moistens and lubricates the cartilage surfaces in the joint. (It resembles the color and texture of an egg white.)

   F. The joint capsule is surrounded by muscles.

   G. The knee joint is a synovial joint that has several bursae to assist with the smooth gliding movement of the tendons as they move over bony parts, or other tendons. A bursa is a small pouch with an inner lining of synovial membrane. It is connected to the synovial membrane of a near-by joint cavity. The bursae contains synovial fluid, which allows it to have a cushioning effect between tissues that rub against one another.

3. **The joint capsule** of the knee is relatively thin, but it is greatly strengthened by ligaments and tendons of several muscles.

4. **Separating the articulating surfaces of the femur and tibia are two menisci, the medial and the lateral meniscus. Each meniscus is somewhat C-shaped.**

TOPIC: KNEE (Continued)

5. Knee injuries:

A. Tearing or displacing a meniscus. This usually occurs when the knee is forcefully twisted, and when the leg is flexed. Since the meniscus is composed of fibrocartilage, such an injury is likely to heal very slowly. Also, if a torn and displaced portion of cartilage becomes jammed between the articulating surfaces, the normal movement of the joint can be hindered.

B. Acute Synovitis. Following an injury to the knee, the synovial membrane may become inflamed (acute synovitis), causing it to secrete an excessive amount of synovial fluid. As a result, the joint cavity soon becomes distended, and the knee begins to look swollen.

C. Fracture of the knee joint can result in loss of joint movement, instability, or the development of arthritis.

6. Disorders of joints:

A. **Dislocation:** Involves the displacement of the articulating bones of a joint. This condition usually occurs as a result of a fall or some other unusual body movement. There is an obvious deformity of the dislocated joint. Some loss of ability to move the body part involved, localized pain, and swelling are symptoms. Medical attention is required for this severe physical problem.

B. **Sprains:** The result of overstretching or tearing the connective tissues, ligaments, and tendons associated with a joint, but without dislocating the articular bones. Sprains are usually caused by forceful wrenching or twisting movements. A sprained joint is likely to bepainful and swollen, and movement at the joint may be restricted. The immediate treatment for a sprain is rest.

C. **Bursitis:** An inflammation of a bursa that maybe caused by excessive use of a joint or by stress on a bursa. The most common initial treatment for bursitis is rest.

D. **Arthritis:** A condition that causes inflamed, swollen and painful joints. There are several types of arthritis, but the most common types are rheumatoid arthritis and osteoarthritis.

1. **Rheumatoid arthritis (RA)** is a painful and potentially crippling disease. In this disease, the synovial membrane of the joint becomes inflamed, and grows thicker. The joint movement becomes increasingly limited, and the articulating bones of the joint may become fused together.

TOPIC: KNEE (Continued)

2. **Osteoarthritis** is the most common type of arthritis. In this condition, the articular cartilages soften and disintegrate gradually, so that the articular surfaces become roughened. It is a common disorder of the aging process. It is likely to affect joints that have received the greatest use over a person's lifetime, such as fingers, hips and knees. The chance of getting osteoarthritis is increased by injury and excess body weight. It usually develops slowly, and it's symptoms can usually be controlled by medication. In severe cases where the joint function is disrupted, parts of the joint may need to be surgically replaced.

E. **Chondromalacia patellae** is a painful disorder of the knee in which the cartilage directly behind the kneecap is damaged. The smooth cartilage over the distal end of the femur, and the inside of the patella, become roughened and no longer glides smoothly. It is painful when the knee is straightened, and when going up stairs. Surgery may be necessary.

F. **A torn menisci can lead to surgery**. Meniscus tears frequently occur where there is not an adequate blood supply to promote healing. When surgery is required, delay could lead to rapid arthritic changes in the knee joint.

7. **Arthroscopy:** Diagnostic arthroscopies are direct internal joint visualization, done by the physician. Arthroscopies are performed in an operating room, under local anesthesia, with an arthroscope. **Diagnostically, this is usually an outpatient procedure. The physician may also do surgical repairs during the course of the arthroscopy.**

8. **Common IDC-9 Codes:**

    836.60..........................Dislocation of knee

    715.00..........................Osteoarthritis

TOPIC: LOWER LEG, ANKLE AND FOOT

1. **The bones of the lower leg are the tibia and the fibula.**

2. **The tibia articulates with the femur.** The tibia is a weight bearing bone and part of the knee joint. It is easily injured because it has little muscle protecting it's anterior surface. Fractures often occur in the middle or distal third, where the circulation is poor. This makes healing difficult.

3. **The tibia and the fibula are frequently broken at the same time, at the distal end, in the area of the malleolus.** (There is a malleolus at the distal end of both the tibia and fibula.) This fracture is called a **Pott's Fracture**. With this fracture the ankle and foot are dislocated outward and backward. Loss of range of motion and loss of weight bearing are two main areas of potential disability.

4. **The ankle is composed of 7 tarsal bones.**

5. **The instep is composed of 5 metatarsal bones.**

6. **The toes are composed of 14 phalanx, or are called the phalanges.**

7. **The Talus and the Calcaneus are frequently injured.** They are both weight bearing bones of the ankle joint. A fractured calcaneus is extremely painful. The Achilles tendon tends to pull the calcaneus from it's usual position, creating a delay in proper healing of the fracture.

8. **The calcaneus fracture is often called an avulsion fracture.** This means that the calcaneus has literally been torn away from it's usual position.

9. **The metatarsals and phalanges are frequently broken when things are dropped on the foot.** They generally heal well with little loss in range of motion.

10. **The most common ankle injury is the inversion sprain.** (A sprain is a ligament tear.) These usually occur when the adducted foot strikes the ground. Inversion sprain symptoms are most often located on the lateral side of the ankle. Symptoms include pain, swelling, and discoloration.

11. **Ankle injuries are common and often minor.** They can, however, lead to recurrent instability, and prolonged disability.

12. **Diagnostic X-rays** (AP and lateral views) are done when the physician suspects a fracture.

13. **The emphasis in treatment of ankle sprains is rest, ice, compression, elevation (RICE).**

14. **RICE and DIETS therapies for ankle injuries:**

    RICE..........................Rest, Ice, Compression, Elevation

    DIETS.......................Drugs*, Injections Exercise Therapy, Surgery
    *Drugs include nonsteroidal anti-inflammatory drugs to reduce pain and inflammation.

61

Joints of the Trunk and Lower Extremity

Pelvis

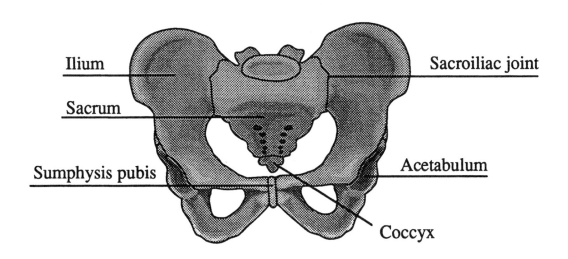

Ilium — — Sacroiliac joint

Sacrum

Sumphysis pubis — — Acetabulum

— Coccyx

Urinary System

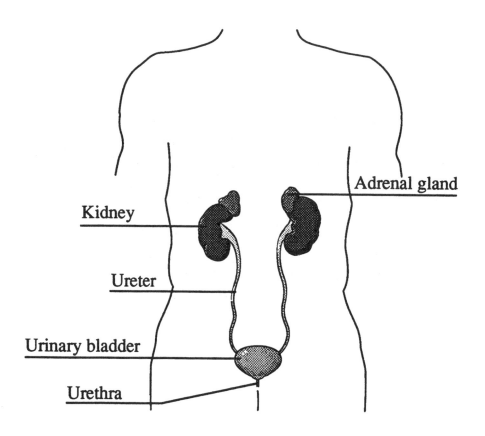

Kidney

Adrenal gland

Ureter

Urinary bladder

Urethra

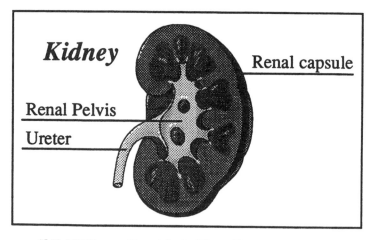

Kidney

Renal capsule

Renal Pelvis

Ureter

"LifeART Images Copyright © 1991 by TechPool Studios, Inc."

Joints of the Trunk and Lower Extremity

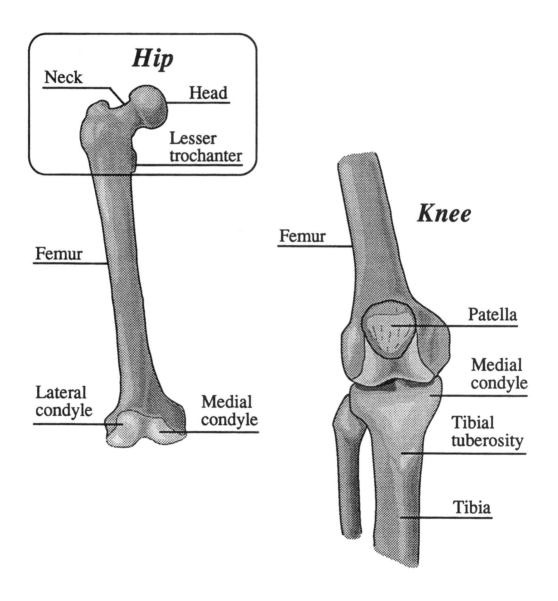

Flexed Knee

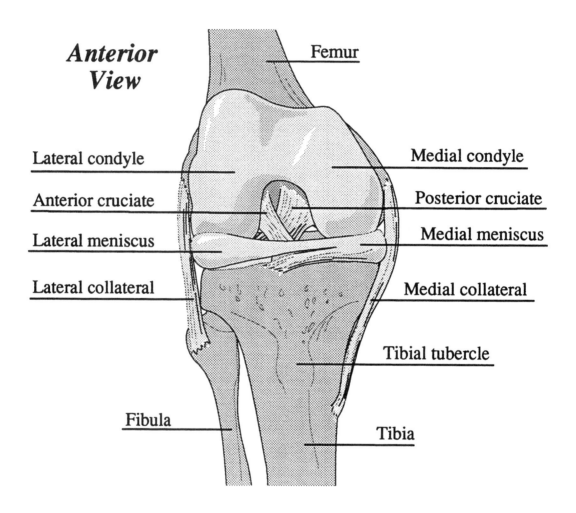

Anterior View

Femur

Lateral condyle

Medial condyle

Anterior cruciate

Posterior cruciate

Lateral meniscus

Medial meniscus

Lateral collateral

Medial collateral

Tibial tubercle

Fibula

Tibia

Medial Knee Joint

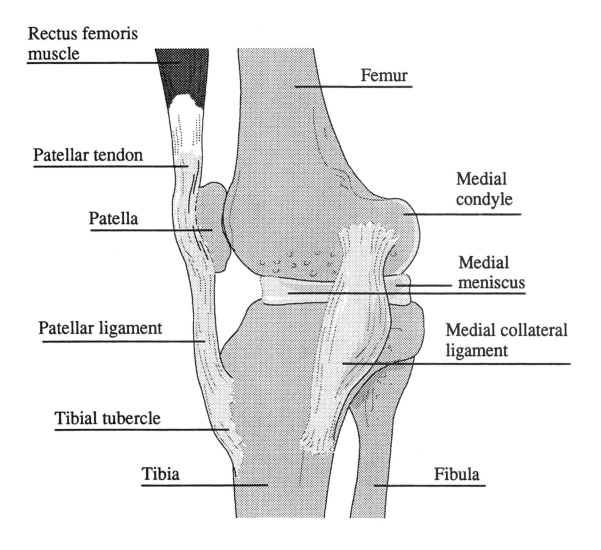

Rectus femoris muscle

Femur

Patellar tendon

Medial condyle

Patella

Medial meniscus

Patellar ligament

Medial collateral ligament

Tibial tubercle

Tibia

Fibula

Joints of the Trunk and Lower Extremity

Ankle

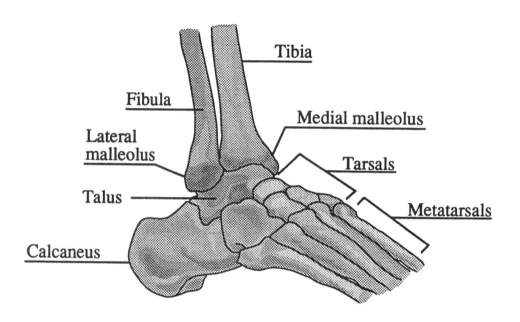

Tibia

Fibula

Medial malleolus

Lateral malleolus

Tarsals

Talus

Metatarsals

Calcaneus

Foot

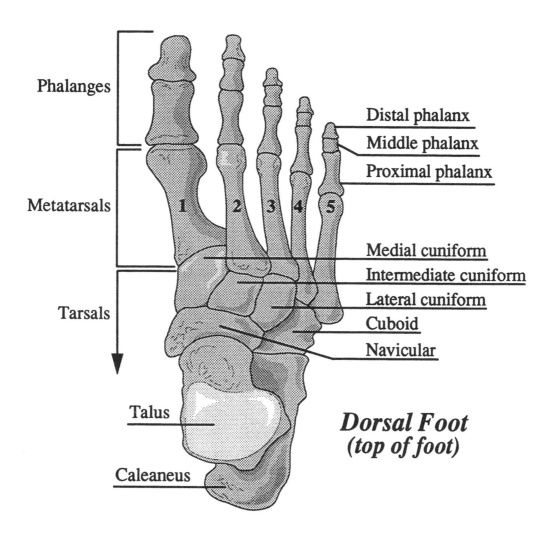

Phalanges

Distal phalanx

Middle phalanx

Proximal phalanx

Metatarsals

1   2   3   4   5

Medial cuniform

Intermediate cuniform

Lateral cuniform

Tarsals

Cuboid

Navicular

Talus

Dorsal Foot
(top of foot)

Caleaneus

Open Book Quiz:

Name: Kim Dabacan

Session: 3

1. What is the acetabulum?

   Is a cavity that the head of the
   Femur Fits into the Pelvis

2. Name 2 bones that articulate with the femur.

   1. Patella - 2. Tibia
   The Lateral + medial condyles.

3. Name the largest ankle bone. It forms the base of what commonly known part of the foot?

   The Calcaneus (heel Bone) - Below the Talus
   Forming the Base of the heel.

4. Where do "hip" fractures commonly occur?

   at the femoral head, neck + acetabulum.

5. What is the difference between the patella and meniscus in the knee?

   Patella - The knee cap - a Flat Bone on the anterior
   surface of the knee
   meniscus - is composed of fibrocartilage.

6. What is synovial fluid? Where is it found?

   Synovial Fluid moistens + lubricates the cartilage
   surfaces in the joint.
   Found in the joints

7. What is a sprain?

   It's caused by overstretching or tearing of the tissues,
   ligaments, and tendons associated with a joint.

8. Describe what happens with a inversion sprain of the ankle.

   pain swelling, + discoloration

9. What does RICE stand for? Why would a doctor order RICE?

   Rest, Ice, compression + Elevation.

10. What is a bursa? What is it's function?

    ~~excessive use of joint~~
    a small pouch with an inter lining of
    synovial membrane.
    — to cushion between tissues that runs together

69

Medical Basics

Chapter 4

TOPIC: MUSCLES   (MY-MYO = MUSCLE)

1. **Muscles are the organs of the muscular system.** Each muscle is composed of cells that are specialized to undergo contraction and relaxation. They are responsible for:

   A. **Movement:** When muscle cells contract, they pull on the body part to which they're attached. This usually causes movement, as with the legs when walking.

   B. **Postural positions:** resist motion, as when holding the body erect, or raising an arm.

   C. **Internal transportation of fluids:** Responsible for the movement of body fluids such as blood and urine.

   D. **Body heat:** They function in heat production, helping to maintain the body's temperature.

2. **There are approximately 600 skeletal muscles in the human body.**

3. **There are 3 types of muscle tissue: skeletal, smooth, cardiac**

   A. **Skeletal:** 40-45 percent of the body weight. By contracting and relaxing, they move bones and joints. They also help maintain body posture.

   Skeletal muscles may be massive like the **gluteus maximus** in the buttock, or as minute as the muscles responsible for facial expressions.

   They are made up of long cells that form bundles. They are controlled by the voluntary nervous system. Skeletal muscles can contract and relax rapidly, but can be easily fatigued.

   B. **Smooth:** Smooth muscles are found surrounding blood vessels, in the iris of the eye, goose bumps, bladder, uterus, fallopian tubes.

   They also are made of long cells that form bundles, but they are under the control of the autonomic nervous system. The circular inner layer produces constriction, and the outer longitudinal layer produces wave-like peristalsis. Smooth muscle contraction is involuntary, as in the intestine.

   C. **Cardiac:** Cardiac muscle is made of short branching cells that form spiral, thick bands of muscle that wrap around the ventricles of the heart. It is also controlled by the autonomic nervous system. Cardiac muscle is also called the myocardium, and is found only in the heart.

TOPIC: MUSCLES

4. **Muscle names are derived from 6 characteristics:**

>   **Action** ....flexion or extension (flexor or extensor)
>
>   **Location** ....for example, near the tibia (tibial muscle)
>
>   **Shape** ....for example, square or triangle (quadrate or deltoid)
>
>   **Points of attachment** ....sternum and mastoid (sternocleidomastoid)
>
>   **Fiber direction** ....as in oblique
>
>   **Number of divisions** ....(biceps or triceps)

Connective Tissue Coverings:

1. **Individual skeletal muscles are separated from adjacent muscles and held in position by layers of fibrous connective tissue called fascia.** This connective tissue surrounds each muscle and may project beyond the end of it's muscle fibers to form a cord-like tendon. The tendon fibers intertwine with the fibers in a bone's periosteum, to attach the muscle to the bone.

2. **Although muscle fibers and the connective tissues associated with them are flexible, they can be torn if they are overstretched.** This creates the common injury of a muscle strain or muscle pull. The seriousness of the injury depends on the degree of damage sustained by the tissues. In a mild strain, for example, only a few muscle fibers are injured, the fascia remains intact, and there is little loss of function. In a severe strain, many muscle fibers as well as fascia are torn, and muscle function may be lost completely. A severe strain is very painful and is accompanied by discoloration and swelling of tissue due to rupture of blood vessels. Such an injury may require surgery to reconnect the separated tissues.

Compartment Syndrome

1. **The space occupied by a particular group of muscles, blood vessels, and nerves, all tightly enclosed by relatively inelastic fascia, constitutes a compartment.** There are many such spaces in the arms and legs. If an injury causes fluid, such as blood from an internal hemorrhage, to accumulate within a compartment, the pressure in the compartment will rise. The increased pressure, in turn, may interfere with blood flow into the region, thus reducing the supply of oxygen and nutrients to the affected tissues. This condition, called compartment syndrome, often produces severe, unrelenting pain, and if the compartmental pressure remains elevated, the enclosed muscles and nerves may be irreversibly damaged.

2. **Treatment for this condition** may involve making a surgical incision through the fascia (fasciotomy) to relieve the excessive pressure and restore the circulation of blood.

TOPIC: MUSCLES VOCABULARY

1. **Contracture:** A condition in which there is a permanent muscular contraction. Can be due to spasm, fibrosis, or paralysis.

2. **Convulsion:** The involuntary contraction of muscles.

3. **Electromyography:** A technique for recording the electrical changes occurring in muscle tissue.

4. **Fibrillation:** Spontaneous contractions of individual muscle fibers, producing rapid and uncoordinated activity within a muscle.

5. **Fibrosis:** A degenerative disease in which skeletal muscle tissue is replaced by fibrous connective tissue.

6. **Fibrositis:** An inflammatory condition of fibrous connective tissues, especially in the muscle fascia. Fibrositis is a term applied to pain and stiffness in the muscles around joints. It is not recognized as a medical term by all medical professionals due to the lack of objective findings. It is sometimes called muscular rheumatism.

7. **Muscular Dystrophy:** A progressively crippling disease of unknown cause in which the muscles gradually weaken and atrophy.

8. **Myalgia:** Pain resulting from any muscular disease or disorder.

9. **Myoma:** A tumor composed of muscle tissue.

10. **Myopathy:** Any muscular disease.

11. **Paralysis:** Loss of voluntary movement in a muscle through injury or disease of the nerve supply.

12. **Paresis:** A partial or slight paralysis of the muscles.

13. **Shin splints:** A nonspecific diagnosis that refers to tenderness and pain in the front of the lower leg. Usually occurs following athletic overexertion.

14. **Torticollis:** A condition in which the neck muscles, such as the sternocleidomastoids, contract involuntarily. It's more commonly called wryneck.

15. **Rheumatism:** A general term for acute and chronic conditions characterized by stiff muscles and pain in joints.

TOPIC: JOINTS

1. **Joints are the junctions between bones of the skeletal system.**

2. **Vocabulary:**

Ankylosis	Loss of mobility of a joint.
Arthrogram	X-ray film of a joint after an injection of radio-paque fluid has been injected into the joint cavity.
Arthroplasty	Surgery performed to make a joint more movable.
Arthroscopy	Examination of the interior of a joint using an instrument called an arthroscope.
Arthrostomy	Surgical opening of a joint to allow fluid drainage
Arthrotomy	Surgical incision of a joint.
Hemarthrosis	Blood in a joint cavity.
Luxation	Dislocation of a joint.
Subluxation	Partial dislocation of a joint.
Synovectomy	Surgical removal of the synovial membrane.

3. **There are 3 types of joints:**

Fibrous	Little or no movement (Skull).
Cartilaginous	Held together by a layer of cartilage (pubis).
Synovial	More complex type of joint (Knee).

4. **Examples of synovial joints are: shoulder, elbow, hip, knee.**

5. **Terms of movement (in addition to the ones already learned):**

Dorsiflexion	Flexing the foot at the ankle (bending the foot upward).
Plantar flexion	Extending the foot at the ankle .
Eversion	Turning the foot so the sole is outward.
Inversion	Turning the foot so the sole is inward.

6. **A sprain is an injury to the ligaments around a joint.** It is the most common injury to a joint. It can involve any joint, but the ankle and wrist are the most frequent sites of sprains. The injury occurs when a sharp sudden twisting movement forces the joint beyond it's normal limits. As a result the ligament may be stretched so much that it tears.

TOPIC: CONDITIONS THAT MAY PROLONG RECOVERY FROM AN INJURY

1. **Osteoporosis is a word meaning porous bone.** It is a condition in which the density of the bone decreases, and brittleness increases. It affects 20 million Americans each year.

   These are primarily post menopausal women and older adults of both sexes. Hip fractures and fractures of the distal forearm are the most common fractures seen with this condition.

   The first symptom of osteoporosis is usually a fracture following a fall that would not normally cause a fracture. Bone loss to osteoporosis can be minimized through exercise and adequate calcium intake.

2. **Multiple Sclerosis (M.S.) is a progressive disease of the central nervous system** (The CNS is composed of the brain and spinal cord). It is a major cause of chronic disability in young adults. It is more common in women (3:2) than men. It's cause is unknown.

   It is thought to be an autoimmune disease in which the body's defense system begins to treat the myelin that covers the nerves as foreign. The body gradually destroys the myelin, causing scarring, and damage to the underlying nerve fibers. M.S. is characterized by transient attacks of weakness, blurred or double vision, slurred speech, and unsteadiness. There is no cure, and treatment is focused on treatment of symptoms.

3. **Muscular Dystrophy:** This is a group of similar congenital muscle disorders leading to increased muscle weakness and paralysis.

4. **Myasthenia Gravis:** A disorder or disease in which the nerve impulses have faulty transmission between the nerve endings and muscles. It usually affects the muscles innervated by the cranial nerves, but can affect other areas as well.

5. **Lupus is a chronic disease that causes inflammation of the connective tissue.** It is an autoimmune disorder in which the body's immune system, for unknown reasons, attacks the connective tissue as though it were foreign, causing inflammation. It is more common in women than men (9:1). The symptoms can be transient.

   The variety called S.L.E. (systemic lupus erythematosus) can affect many systems of the body, including the joints and kidneys. Symptoms of S.L.E. can include minor things like a red rash over the cheeks and nose, a feeling of illness, fever; to more major symptoms like loss of appetite, arthritis, pericarditis, and renal failure.

6. **Osteomyelitis:** A bone or bone marrow inflammation. It usually stems from bacterial infection (staphlococcus). It may, however, be caused by fungus, paracites, and viruses.

TOPIC: CONDITIONS THAT MAY PROLONG RECOVERY FROM AN INJURY (Continued)

7. **Osteoarthritis is the most common type of arthritis.** In this condition, the articular cartilages soften and disintegrate gradually, so that the articular surfaces become roughened.

   It's a common disorder of the aging process. It is likely to affect the joints that have received the greatest use over a person's lifetime, such as the fingers, hips and knees.

   Chances of getting this disorder are increased by injury and excess body weight.

8. **ICD-9 codes common to muscles and joints:**

   729.1....................Myalgia and myositis
   (pain in muscle and inflammation of muscle tissue)

   728.85 ....Spasm muscle

   728.2....................Fibrositis
   (inflammation of white, fibrous connective tissue)

   836.60 ....Dislocation Knee

   727.05 ....Tendonitis Wrist

   845.00 ....Sprain/strain Ankle

   727.2....................Bursitis

   715.00 ....Osteoarthritis

Skeletal System

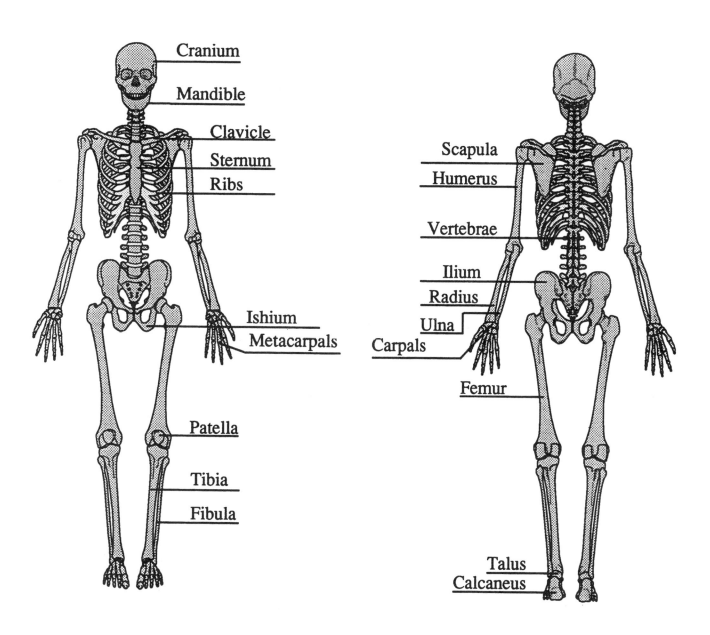

Cranium
Mandible
Clavicle
Sternum
Ribs
Ishium
Metacarpals
Patella
Tibia
Fibula

Scapula
Humerus
Vertebrae
Ilium
Radius
Ulna
Carpals
Femur
Talus
Calcaneus

There are 206 bones in the human skeleton. These are divided into two categories. The *axial* skeleton has 74 bones (forming the upright axis of the body) plus 6 tiny bones in the middle ear. The *apendicular* skeleton has the 126 bones of the shoulder, hip, arms and legs.

Skeletal Muscles

need to know these?

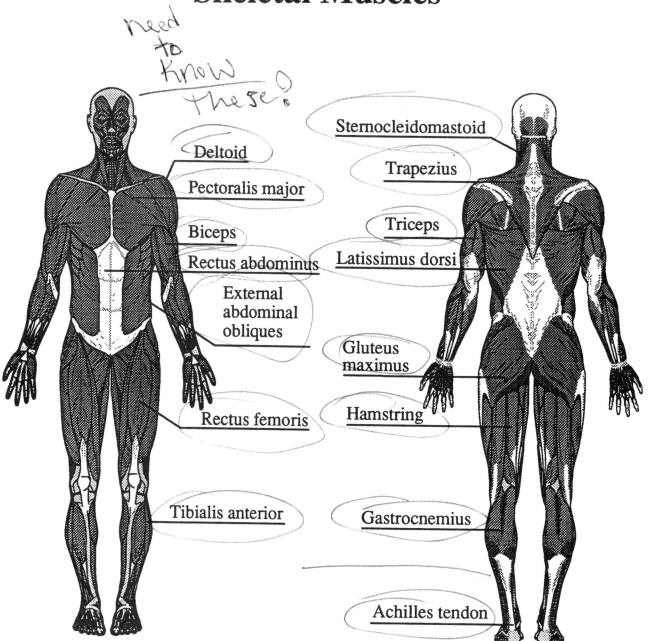

Deltoid

Pectoralis major

Biceps

Rectus abdominus

External abdominal obliques

Rectus femoris

Tibialis anterior

Sternocleidomastoid

Trapezius

Triceps

Latissimus dorsi

Gluteus maximus

Hamstring

Gastrocnemius

Achilles tendon

There are more than 600 skeletal muscles in the human body.
These muscles attach to bone, connective tissue, soft tissue, or skin.
They help produce movement, maintain posture, and generate heat.

Medical Basics

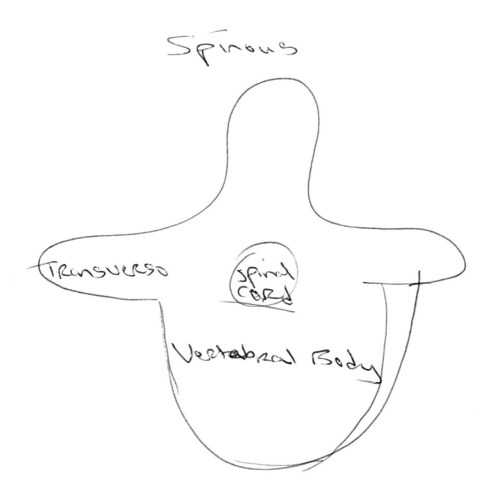

Spinous

Transverso

Spinal Cord

Vertebral Body

TOPIC: THE SPINE   (Vertebral Column)

The spine is composed of 33 vertebrae: 7 cervical, 12 thoracic, 5 lumbar, a sacrum composed of 5 fused segments, and a coccyx composed of 4 fused segments.

1. **Cervical vertebrae (7)**

    The Atlas, or 1st cervical vertebra, supports and balances the head. It is joined to the Axis, or 2nd cervical vertebra. The Axis has a tooth-like projection that projects upward, and lies in the ring of the Atlas. This is the odontoid process. When the head turns, the atlas pivots around the odontoid process.

    These are the smallest vertebrae. Their bone tissue is denser than that in any other area of the spine.

2. **Thoracic vertebrae (12) are often called the dorsal vertebrae.**

    They increase with size as they move downward. This adapts them to the increasing amounts of body weight placed on them.

    They are unique because of their rib attachments on each side. These facets (facet = small smooth area on a bone) are called the costal pits.

    Injury is less frequent in the thoracic area because of the support given by the ribs.

3. **Lumbar vertebrae (5)**

    They located in the small of the back.

    They have larger, stronger bodies, enabling them to support more weight.

    These are the most commonly injured vertebrae

4. **Sacrum (5 fused vertebrae)**

    The vertebrae develop separately, but then fuse into one

    The sacrum articulates with the hip at the ilium, forming the sacroiliac joint. The weight of the body is transmitted to the legs through the pelvic girdle at these joints.

5. **Coccyx (4 fused vertebrae)**

    These develop separately. The vertebrae fuse into one by early adulthood.

    The coccyx is commonly called the tail bone.

    It is attached to the sacrum by ligaments. This gives it a minor degree of flexibility, allowing it to move slightly forward during the act of sitting.

TOPIC: VERTEBRAE

Structure:

The **vertebral body** is the anterior portion of the vertebra. It is an oval, solid segment of bone.

There are two **transverse processes** that stick out on each side of the vertebrae.
The **spinous process** is in the middle.

      a.   The bony plates that fuse to form the process are called **laminae.**

      b.   The laminae are flattened plates of bone on either side of the arch of a vertebra.

      c.   Other processes are the **articular processes** that allow movement between two vertebrae

The **vertebral foramen** is the opening that allows passage of the spinal cord.

TOPIC: LIGAMENTS

There are many ligaments involved in the structure of the spine.
Two of the most important ligaments are:

The **anterior longitudinal ligament** extends from the Atlas to the sacrum. It binds the disks with the margins of the vertebra.

The **posterior longitudinal ligament** lies on the posterior surface of the bodies of the vertebrae. It extends from the Axis to the sacrum.

Vocabulary:

Kyphosis ....is an exaggeration of the normal posterior curve of the spine. It is called "hump back" in common usage.

Lordosis ....is an abnormal anterior convexity of the spine, giving the lower spine a forward curve. It is called "sway back" in common usage.

Scoliosis ....is a lateral curvature of the spine.

TOPIC: THE INTERVERTEBRAL DISK

1. By definition, the intervertebral disk is the fibrocartilaginous tissue between the vertebral bodies.

2. The intervertebral disk:

Acts as a cushion between the bony surfaces of the vertebral bodies.

Helps allow the vertebrae greater motion.

Helps distribute weight over a large surface during movement.

Acts as a shock absorber.

The disk's outside is called the annulus fibrosus.

The middle of the disk is called the nucleus pulposus. It is composed of collagen fibrils that produce an elastic central mass. It's high water content decreases with age.

Both the annulus fibrosus and the nucleus pulposus are without blood supply in the adult.

3. Herniated disk:

Increasing age brings on degenerative changes:

    The nucleus pulposus loses it's firmness.

    The annulus fibrosus becomes thinner, weaker, and develops small cracks.

    DDD is the abbreviation used for degenerative disk disease.

A herniated (ruptured or prolapsed) disk occurs when the little cracks, combined with the pressure brought on by a fall or lifting a heavy object, cause the outer layer of the disk to break. When the central mass squeezes out through the crack, the disk is said to have herniated.

A herniation can occur at any level, but most commonly occurs with the lumbar disks.

Herniated disks are most common between the ages of 30-40. After the age of 40, extra fibrous tissue forms around the disks, increasing their stability.

TOPIC: TERMS

Ankylosing spondylitis ....is an inflammatory disease of the spine which leads to bony ankylosis of the vertebral articulations. (**Ankylosis** is immobility and fixation of a joint.)

Arachnoiditis ....is inflammation of the arachnoid tissue. It can lead to fibrosis that binds the roots of the cauda equina.

Degenerative disk disease (DDD) ....is a condition in which the deterioration of a disk produces clinical symptoms and signs.

Disk degeneration ....is the loss of the structural and functional integrity of the disk.

Herniated nucleus pulposus ....is the displacement of the nucleus pulposus material beyond the confines of the annulus.

Interspinous pseudarthrosis ....is the development of a false joint between two spinous processes.

Pseudarthrosis ....is the failure of union in either bone or bone graft.

Radiculitis ....is the inflammation of a spinal nerve.

Radiculopathy ....is a non-inflammatory abnormality of a spinal nerve in the spinal canal or neural foramen resulting in neurological deficit.

Spinal stenosis ....is the reduction in the size of the spinal canal, to a point that causes cord compression. There are two types:

    Congenital/developmental ....present at birth or genetic.

    Acquired stenosis ....through trauma or surgery.

Spondylitis ....is an inflammatory disease of the spine.

Spondylolisthesis ....is the anterior displacement (slipping forward) of the top vertebrae of two adjacent vertebra. A common site is L-5, S-1. It can develop in several ways:

    Degenerative..........................caused by degenerative changes that erode the vertebral joints.

    Traumatic ....anterior displacement of a vertebra due to traumatic injury to it's restraining structures.

    Pathologic ....anterior displacement of a vertebra due to a disease process in the bone.

Spondylosis ....is a degenerative disease of both the disc and vertebra. It may cause pressure on nerve roots, if severe.

Medical Basics

Medical Basics — Chapter 5

TOPIC: SURGICAL TERMS

Discectomy — is the removal of all or part of a disk.

Discography — is a diagnostic test where radiopaque fluid is injected into the nucleus pulposus for purposes of identifying the shape of the disk.

Spinal fusion — is the joining of two or more vertebrae.

Hemilaminectomy — is the removal of one half of a lamina.

Internal fixation — is the union of two or more vertebrae with implants of metal.

Laminectomy — is the removal of a lamina.

Laminotomy — is creating an opening in a lamina.

Neurolysis — is the separation of a nerve from adhering scar tissue.

TOPIC: TESTS AND SIGNS

Babinski toe sign — When stroking the sole of the foot, the big toe will either go up (a positive sign, indicating nerve loss), or go down (a negative sign, or normal response).

Leseques sign — is a straight leg raising test for sciatica. With the patient supine, the extended leg is raised from the table. The test is positive if the leg can't be raised to 80-90 degrees without sciatica pain.

Marxer test — is an indication of functional behavior when the patient complains of sciatic pain when the prone patient's knee's are flexed slightly.

Waddel signs — is the signs and tests that indicate a functional, hysterical, or malingering patient. The presence of any three of the following symptoms usually indicates that surgical treatment will fail:

non organic tenderness, non-anatomic sensory loss, collapsing, give-away weakness, or interference with the examination.

TOPIC: SPINAL TRAUMA TERMS

Dislocation ....is a complete loss of contact of the articular surfaces of a joint.

Fracture ....is a disruption in the continuity of a bone.

Lumbosacral sprain ....is a ligamentous injury of the lumbosacral region.

Lumbosacral strain ....is a musculature injury of the lumbosacral region.

Subluxation ....is partial loss of contact of the articulating surfaces of bone.

TOPIC: CLINICAL TERMS

Intermittent claudication ......is the description of complaints of leg pain and lameness, brought on by walking. It is usually caused by ischemia of the muscles used in walking, and may have a vascular origin.

Lumbago ....is low back pain with or without radiation into the buttock and posterior thigh.

Sciatica ....is pain along the course of the sciatic nerve.

Thoracic outlet syndrome ......is neurovascular dysfunction in the upper limb arising from compression of the subclavian vessels and/or the brachial plexus at the base of the neck.

A trigger point ....is any place on the body that, when stimulated, results in pain being referred to a predictable area on the skin. The area of referral can be a distance away from the trigger point. For example, when the trigger point of the extensor carpi radialis is stimulated, sensation should be felt over the dorsum of the hand.

TOPIC: SPINAL CORD

1. **The spinal cord begins at the lower portion of the brain stem (the medulla oblongata), and extends to approximately L-2.**

2. **It is covered by the same 3 layers of meninges that cover the brain.**

3. **It is composed of nerve rich tissue.** Out of this tissue comes all the nerves to the trunk and limbs of the body.

4. **The spinal cord is responsible for:**

    All nerve impulses that occur in the body with the exception of the head.

    All reflex action, action that does not require thought for a response.

5. **The spinal cord doesn't take up all the space in the vertebral foramina.**
    The three protective meninges are there in addition to the cerebrospinal fluid.

    The cerebrospinal fluid is located between the arachnoid and pia mater in the subarachnoid space.

    Cerebrospinal fluid is also found in the brain.

    It's function is to form a water cushion protection for the brain and spinal cord, protecting it from physical impact.

TOPIC: SPINAL NERVES

1. **There are 31 pair of nerves originating in the spinal cord.** Most of them have no special names, but are numbered according to the level where they emerge from the spinal column.

2. The cervical and thoracic nerves branch out horizontally, but the lumbar, sacral and coccygeal nerves descend to the lower end of the cord forming the **cauda equina (horses tail)**.

3. Each spinal nerve emerges from the cord by two short branches, or roots, which lie in the vertebral column.

4. The area of skin innervated by various spinal nerves is called a **dermatome.**

TOPIC: SPINAL CORD INJURY

The spinal cord is the main communication route between the CNS and the rest of the body. When it's injured, the whole body may be affected.

The spinal cord may be injured indirectly, as in a blow to the head or a fall, or by direct injury to the surrounding vertebrae. The consequences will depend on the amount of damage sustained by the cord.

In minor injuries to the spinal cord, as in whiplash from an automobile accident, or with the rupture of a disk, the cord may be compressed or distorted. Such injuries are often accompanied by **pain, weakness,** and **muscular atrophy** in the regions supplied by the damaged nerve fibers. These symptoms can often be alleviated through treatment.

Among the more common causes of severe direct injury to the spinal cord are gunshot wounds, stabbings, and fractures and dislocations that can occur during automobile accidents. With a severe traumatic injury, the vertebrae can be damaged through dislocation, fracture, or rupture of the ligaments that bind them together. In these cases, bone, accumulated fluid, or a blood clot may press on the cord. The cord may be torn or severed. In any of these situations, the function of the cord is impaired, or may even be destroyed.

When there is pressure on the spinal cord, surgery to remove the source of the pressure may bring improvement in the symptoms. Even when there is minor damage to the cord, some improvement may occur up to 12 months following the injury.

The vertebra injured in a severe cord injury, relates to the following probable level of permanent recovery:

C1 to C4	Quadriplegia with respiratory function impairment.
C5 to C6	Quadriplegia with some control of shoulders.
C6 to T1	"Low quad", more use of arms and trunk.
T1 to T2	Paraplegia, torso balance improved.
T3 to T12	Paraplegia, wheelchair independence.
L1 to L2	"Low Para", with possible walking with brace and cane.
L3 to L4	Para..but walking is possible. May have foot drop. May need a knee brace.

Anatomy

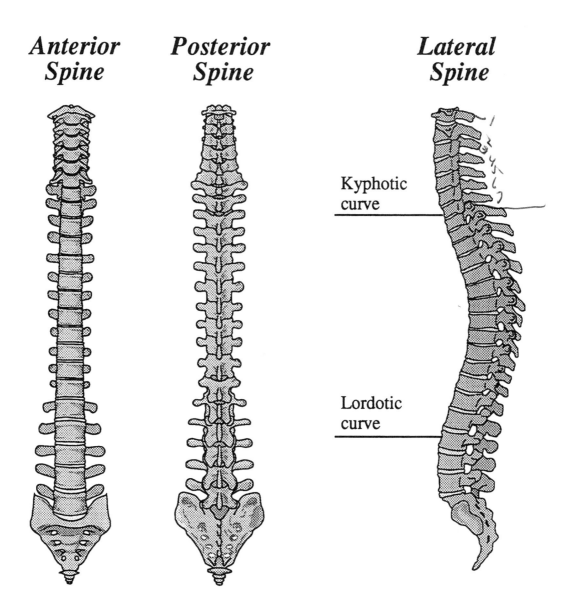

Anterior Spine   **Posterior Spine**   **Lateral Spine**

Kyphotic curve

Lordotic curve

Lordosis: exaggerated lordotic curve in the lumbar area.
Kyphosis: exaggerated kyphotic curve in the upper spine.
Scoliosis: lateral curvature of the spine.

Anatomy

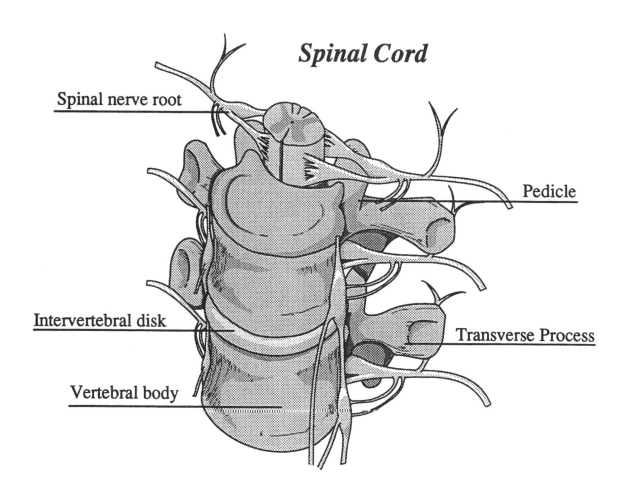

Spinal Cord

Spinal nerve root

Pedicle

Intervertebral disk

Transverse Process

Vertebral body

Open Book Quiz:

Name: Kim Dabacon

Session: 5

1. What happens when a disk herniates?

   The little cracks with pressure - cause the outer layer of the disk to break and the central mass squeezes out the crack.

2. Where does the spinal cord begin and end?

   Begins at the lower part of the brain stem & descends to L-2.

3. What is a subluxed vertebra?

   Is partial loss of contact of the articulating surface of the bone.

4. What happens with a lumbar strain?

   Is a musculature injury of the Lumbosacral region.

5. What happens with a lumbar sprain?

   a ligamentous injury of the Lumbosacral region.

6. What is the portion of a vertebra that allows joint movement?

   There are 2 transverse processes that stick out on eachside of the vertebra - articular processes the movement!

7. What is spinal stenosis? How does a person get it?

   Is the reduction in the size of the spinal canal to a point that causes cord compression. 1. present at birth or genetic - 2. thru trauma or surgery.

8. What is the cauda equina?

   The lumbar, sacral and coccygeal nerves that descend to the lower end of the spinal cord forming the (horses tail)

9. What is a diskectomy? How is it different from a laminectomy?

   Is the removal of a/all or part of a disk.
   Laminectomy is the removal of a lamina.

10. How many pair of spinal nerves are there?

    31 pair

Medical Basics

TOPIC: RESPIRATORY SYSTEM   (PULMO - LUNG)
(PHEUM - TO BREATHE)

1. The respiratory system includes the nose, nasal cavity, sinuses, pharynx, larynx, trachea, bronchial tree, and lungs.

2. The bronchial tree connects the trachea to the alveoli, through it's bronchioles.

3. The alveoli cluster like tiny grapes around the ends of the bronchioles. There are millions of these balloon-like sacs.

4. The alveoli are surrounded by a capillary network from the pulmonary artery and vein. They are responsible for the exchange of oxygen and carbon dioxide in the blood.

5. The lungs are soft, spongy, cone-shaped organs located in the thoracic cavity. They are enclosed by the thoracic cage and the diaphragm.

6. The lungs are covered by the pleural membrane..or pleura. This same membrane lines the inside of the chest cavity...Fluid between the two layers allows for smooth fluid motion during breathing. Pleurisy is inflammation of the pleura.

7. **Diseases of the respiratory system:**

   Reactive airway disease ....is airway reaction to inhaled irritants.

   Asthma ....is recurring bouts of breathlessness, characterized by wheezing when breathing out. It can be either **extrinsic** (usually triggered by something inhaled) or **intrinsic** (where there's no apparent external cause). Asthma has no cure. Treatment consists of preventing attacks, and treating the symptoms when they occur. A bronchodilator is a medication that relaxes and widens the airways.

   Bronchitis ....occurs when the bronchi become inflamed. A bronchospasm occurs when the smoothe muscle in the walls of the bronch constricts, causing a narrowing of the airway.

   Emphysema ....is a disease in which the alveoli of the lungs become damaged. It can cause shortness of breath and heart failure. It can be caused by smoking or atmospheric pollution. It's often accompanied by chronic bronchitis. The two together are called chronic obstructive pulmonary disease (COPD).

TOPIC: RESPIRATORY SYSTEM   (Continued)

Pulmonary embolism ....can result in obstruction of the pulmonary artery or one of it's branches in the lung by an embolus. The embolus is a fragment that has broken off from a blood clot in a vein.

8. **Pulmonary function tests** are a group of procedures used to evaluate the function of the lungs.

9. **The diaphragm** is a large muscle that separates the thorax from the abdominal cavity. It attaches to the spine, the ribs, and the sternum.

10. The diaphragm plays a vital role in breathing:

    As you breathe in, the diaphragm tightens and pulls down, giving the lungs more space. The lungs fill with air. (the rib muscles also tighten, making the ribs move up and out.)

    As you breathe out, the diaphragm relaxes and arches up. (the rib muscles relax and the ribs move down and in. This pushes some of the air out of your lungs.)

11. **Hiccups are a spasm of the diaphragm**, followed by rapid closure of the vocal cords (causing the characteristic hiccup sound).

12. **Hiatal Hernia** is a type of hernia that occurs when a part of the stomach protrudes upward into the chest through a hiatus (opening) in the diaphragm. It's cause is unknown. It occurs most commonly in middle aged women. Obesity and smoking have also been linked to it's incidence.

13. **Vocabulary:**

    Apnea ....a temporary absence of breathing.

    Atelectasis ....collapse of some portion of a lung.

    Dyspnea ....difficulty breathing.

    Tracheotomy ....an incision in the trachea.

    Thoracotomy ....surgical incision of the chest wall.

    Pneumonectomy ......removal of a lung.

    Lobectomy ....removal of a lobe of the lung.

    Bronchoscopy ....diagnostic examination of the bronchi through a bronchoscope.

    Pneumonia ....inflammation of the lung caused primarily by bacteria.

TOPIC: CIRCULATORY SYSTEM

1. The heart and blood vessels compose the circulatory system.
   Another name for this system is the **cardiovascular system.**

2. The circulatory system provides all body tissues with a regular supply of oxygen and nutrients, and carries away carbon dioxide and other waste products.

3. Arteries carry the oxygenated blood to the body.
   Veins return the deoxygenated blood to the heart.

4. The pulmonary circulation circulates through the lungs.
   The portal circulation circulates blood through the liver.

5. The main function of blood is to act as the body's transport system.
   It also plays a major role in the defense against infection.

6. The average adult has about 10 pints of blood. Almost half this volume is cells.
   These are:

red blood cells ....erythrocytes ......RBCs ....carry oxygen
white cells ....leukocytes ....WBCs...............fight against infection
platelets ....thrombocytes............................help in blood clotting

The remainder of the fluid is called plasma. Plasma contains dissolved proteins, sugars, fats, and minerals. It transports waste products of the body to the kidneys. Plasma proteins are a part of the immune system.

TOPIC: HEART   (CARDIA - HEART)

1. The heart is a muscular pump that, throughout life, beats continuously and rhythmically to send blood to the lungs and to the rest of the body. During an average lifetime, the heart contracts more than 2.5 billion times.

2. In one day, the heart beats approximately 100,000 times, and pumps approximately 4,000 gallons of blood, and keeps the blood circulating in about 100,000 miles of arteries, capillaries and veins.

3. Heart structure:

    Myocardium (heart muscle). Given sufficient oxygen and nutrients, it contracts rhythmically and automatically without any other stimulation.

    The interior of the heart consists of four distinct chambers. A thick central muscular wall (**the septum**) divides the cavity into right and left halves. Each half consists of an upper chamber (**atrium**), and a lower chamber (**ventricle**). Various large blood vessels emerge from the top and sides of the heart; they deliver blood to the atria or carry blood pumped out by the ventricles.

    The internal surface of the heart is lined with a smooth membrane...the **endocardium.** The entire heart is enclosed in a tough, membranous bag (**the pericardium**).

    It is protected by the sternum in front, the rib cage and lungs around it, the diaphragm under it, and the spine behind it.

4. The heart is a two sided pump. Each side functions independently, but in unison. Here's what is happening during the heart beat:

    Left Ventricle .... blood is oxygen rich, the ventricle contracts, forcing the blood into the aorta. The aorta carries the oxygenated blood to the body.

    Superior and inferior vena cava ... are veins that transport the deoxygenated blood back from the body into the heart.

    Right Atrium .... collects the oxygen deficient blood, and moves it to the right ventricle.

    Right ventricle .... contracts, sending the blood to the pulmonary artery, to the lungs. (in the lungs, the blood gives up the wastes and carbon dioxide, which are breathed out, and picks up the oxygen that is breathed in.) The pulmonary veins return the oxygenated blood to the heart.

    Left Atrium .... collects the oxygen rich blood, moves it to the left ventricle, and the cycle begins again.

TOPIC: HEART (Continued)

5. The **atrium chambers** are reservoirs to the lower pumping ventricle chambers.

6. The heart has valves that separate each anatomical compartment. They are extremely thin, powerful, and efficient. They work in one direction only, to prevent a backflow of blood.
   Examples:

   aortic valve ....between the ascending aorta and the left ventricle

   bicuspid valve ....(mitral valve) between the left. atrium and left ventricle

   tricuspid valve ....between the right atrium and the right ventricle

   pulmonary valve ....separates the pulmonary artery and
   the right ventricle

7. The rhythm of the heartbeat has the mitral and tricuspid valves opening then closing in unison.

8. The heart's natural pacemaker...the **S-A node**...is located in the wall of the right atrium. The S-A node puts out electric current...that the ventricles receive, making them contract. The contracting of the ventricles is called the heartbeat.

9. Two parts of the heartbeat are:

   diastole ....heart is at rest—that is, when blood from
   the atrium is pouring into the ventricle.

   systole ....is the contraction.

10. The two numbers in a blood pressure reading correspond to the heartbeat phases:

    the **systolic** (or higher number) ......is a measurement of the blood's pressure
    against artery walls when the heart is at work.

    the **diastolic** ....is a measurement of blood pressure during
    the heart's relaxation period.

11. The heart muscle receives it's oxygen and nutrients from the **coronary arteries** on it's surface.

12. The **EKG**...electrocardiogram...is a diagnostic test that traces the heart's electrical current. Among the things it can indicate are irregular heartbeat rhythms and signs of heart muscle damage caused by a blocked coronary artery.

13. **Angiography** is a diagnostic test done with a radioactive dye that allows the doctor to observe and monitor the function of the heart's structure.

14. **Cardiac catheterization...angiocardiography**... is a diagnostic test where a thin, flexible tube is inserted through a blood vessel and on into the heart. The passage of the tube is observed by doctors using fluoroscopy.

TOPIC: ATHEROSCLEROSIS

1. **Atherosclerosis** causes a narrowing of interior portions of arteries. The narrowing occurs in relation to the accumulation of lipids and other substances on the inner wall of the blood vessel. It's presence may be related to age, diet and inherited tendencies.

2. **Atherosclerotic heart disease** involving the coronary arteries is the most common single cause of death in the U.S. Atherosclerotic interference with blood supply to the brain (causing stroke) is the third most common cause of death (cancer is the second).

3. The development of atherosclerosis can be related to some of the following factors:

   cigarette smoking

   hypertension

   male gender (ratio 6:1)

   obesity

   limited physical activity

   high serum cholesterol

   family history of arterial disease

   diabetes

   anxious or aggressive personality (possibly)

   *risk increases with age

4. The accumulations on the interior of the artery are called **plaques.** The word plaque means a raised patch. They are composed of lipids, decaying muscle cells, fibrous tissue, clumps of blood platelets, cholesterol, and sometimes calcium. These cholesterol rich, fatty deposits are called **atheromas.**

5. Plaques tend to form is areas of turbulent blood flow. They are found most often in individuals that have a high cholesterol level.

TOPIC: CORONARY HEART DISEASE (CHD)

1. **Coronary heart disease** is the damage to, or malfunction of, the heart caused by narrowing or blockage of the coronary arteries. The coronary arteries supply blood to the heart muscle.

2. Two manifestations of CHD are:

    Angina pectoris ....(chest pain).

    Myocardial infarction..................(heart attack).

3. CHD causes:

    A reduction in the blood flow to the heart muscle.

    A reduction in the blood flow to the heart's electrical conduction system.

4. The coronary arteries first become narrowed by the plaques, decreasing the amount of blood that flows through them. They may eventually become totally blocked by the atheroma that has formed.

5. A piece of the atheroma may break off...causing it to become a free floater in the blood stream. This is called an **embolus**. It may completely occlude the lumen of a small blood vessel.

6. Coronary heart disease symptoms:

    It is usually asymptomatic in it's early stages.

    The first symptom is usually either angina pectoris or heart attack.

7. Angina pectoris:

    Angina is ....discomfort or pain in the chest that is usually relieved by rest.

    Angina pain is ....a dull ache in the middle of the chest, or a feeling of pressure that may spread up to the neck or down the arms (the left more often than the right).

    It occurs when ....the heart muscle is working hard and getting too little blood for the amount of effort being expended.

TOPIC: CORONARY HEART DISEASE (CHD)   (Continued)

8. If the blood supply to part of the muscle is cut off completely, the result is an acute myocardial infarction…heart attack.

9. **Myocardial Infarction (MI):**

> Many victims of myocardial infarction have a history of angina pectoris. The pain of a MI comes on suddenly, ranges from a tight ache to intense crushing agony. It can last for 30 minutes or more, and is not relieved by rest. Pain is the first symptom of MI.

> The other symptoms may include shortness of breath, restlessness, and the individual may be apprehensive, with cold clammy skin, feel nauseated, and possibly lose consciousness.

> Damage to the heart muscle can cause **arrhythmias** (abnormal heart beat rhythm) and heart failure. Heart failure is failure of the heart to maintain adequate circulation of the blood through failure of it's pumping action.

TOPIC: IMMUNE SYSTEM

1. Immunity is a state of protection against disease through the activities of the immune system. Natural, or innate, immunity is present from birth. Acquired immunity results from exposure to invading microorganism, or as a result of immunizations.

2. The immune system helps protect against infection with the help of **phagocytes.** These are cells capable of surrounding, engulfing, and digesting microorganisms (such as bacteria and viruses, and cellular debris). They are found in the blood, spleen, and lymph nodes, and in the alveoli. Some types of white blood cells (produced in the bone marrow) are phagocytes. These are "free" phagocytes, able to wander through the tissues and engulf organisms and cellular debris at will. This process is called **phagocytosis.**

3. In certain circumstances, such as after transplant, and in people with an autoimmune disorder, the immune system is suppressed by giving autoimmune medication. This is called immunosuppression.

4. Immunosuppression can also occur after infection with certain viruses, including HIV (**human immunodeficiency virus**), the virus that causes AIDS (**acquired immunodeficiency syndrome**).

5. Opportunistic infections are infections that occur in people with immunodeficiency disorders. The microorganisms take advantage of a persons lowered defenses. Common ones are pneumonia, herpes simplex infections, and many fungal infections.

6. **Herpes simplex** is a common viral disease. There are two types.
    There is a considerable overlapping of the two types. Both are contagious:

    HSV1 ....infections of the lips, mouth, and face

    HSV2 ....infections of the genitals and babies at birth
    (genital herpes)

    If a person with AIDS, or someone who is taking immunosuppressive drugs is infected with the virus, it can cause severe general infection that is sometimes fatal.

7. **Herpes Zoster** (shingles) is a viral infection of the nerves that supply certain areas of the skin. It is caused by the same virus that causes chicken-pox. During an attack of the chicken-pox, most of the virus is destroyed. Some of the virus survives, however, and lie dormant in certain sensory nerves..sometimes for many years. When the immune system is compromised by stress or the use of corticosteroid drugs, herpes zoster can appear.

8. **Hepatitis A** is a virus infection, called viral hepatitis. The primary target of this virus is the liver. It is spread from the direct, or indirect contact with human feces from an infected person. This could include form contaminated food, drinking water, or a person's fingers. The symptoms include a flu-like illness with jaundice, usually occurring 3-6 weeks after exposure.

TOPIC: IMMUNE SYSTEM (Continued)

9. **Hepatitis B** is a virus infection called serum hepatitis. Needle sticks and sexual transmission are the primary transmission routes of this disease. Symptoms occur 6 weeks to 6 months after exposure. Vaccines are available to boost immunity for Hepatitis B. B is more serious than A. The virus can persist for many years after the initial infection, and can lead to a chronic form of hepatitis, and other liver diseases. Carriers can be asymptomatic, but still infect others... approximately 5-10 percent become chronic carriers.

10. **AIDS** is a deficiency of the immune system due to infection with HIV. AIDS is a progression of the HIV infection. The immune system is weakened by THe HIV virus, and when disease organisms invade, the body's immune responses may fail. Disease organisms may then overwhelm the immune system. Many infections are more common, or more severe in HIV positive individuals. These infections include herpes simplex, shingles, tuberculosis.

    Full blown AIDS includes cancers, infections, diarrhea, and chronic herpes simplex.

11. Medications such as AZT and acyclovar are antiviral drugs that are sometimes given to help the immunosuppressed patient fight a significant viral infection.

12. Fungal infections are more common and more serious in people who are taking corticosteroid drugs or immunosuppressant drugs, or who are immunosuppressed. They are called opportunistic because they take advantage of an individuals lowered defenses.

13. Surgical infections: Infections following surgery are usually bacterial in origin.
    The 5 classical symptoms of infection are:

    pain

    heat

    redness

    swelling

    disordered function

    Antibiotic treatment is indicated for treatment.

TOPIC: ICD-9 CODES FOR COMMON CONDITIONS

1. **Cardiac:**

   786.50 ....Chest Pain

   410.9...................Myocardial infarction

2. **Vascular:**

   453.9...................Thrombosis (a blood clot)

   904.9...................Injury to a blood vessel

3. **Respiratory:**

   493.90 ....Asthma

   506.0...................Bronchitis, chemical

4. **Immune System:**

   V01.7 ....Exposure to AIDS

Respiratory System

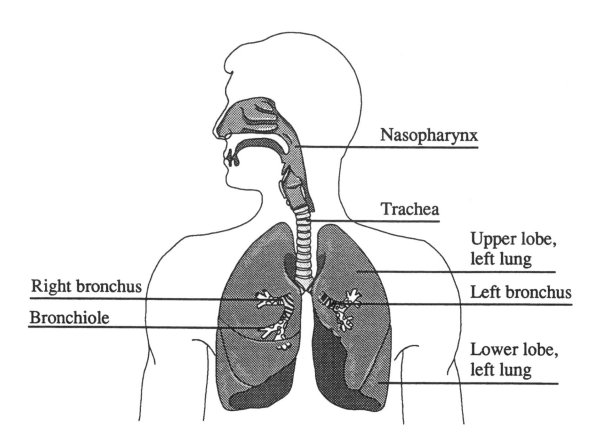

Nasopharynx

Trachea

Upper lobe,
left lung

Right bronchus

Left bronchus

Bronchiole

Lower lobe,
left lung

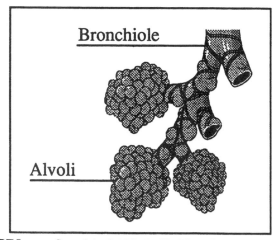

Bronchiole

Alvoli

Fig: 6-B

Blood Cells

White blood cells

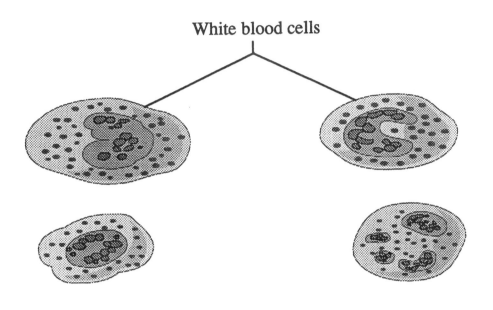

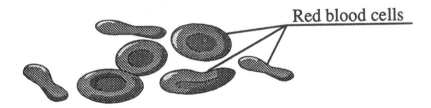

Red blood cells

Arterial Circulation

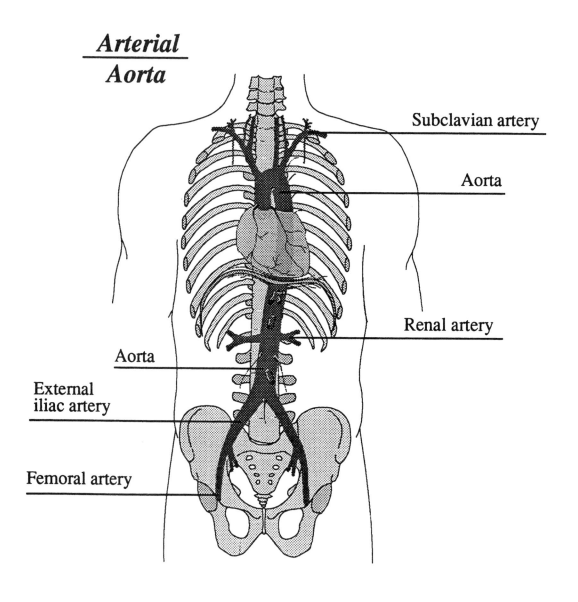

Arterial
Aorta

Subclavian artery

Aorta

Renal artery

Aorta

External
iliac artery

Femoral artery

Fig: 6-D

Venous Circulation

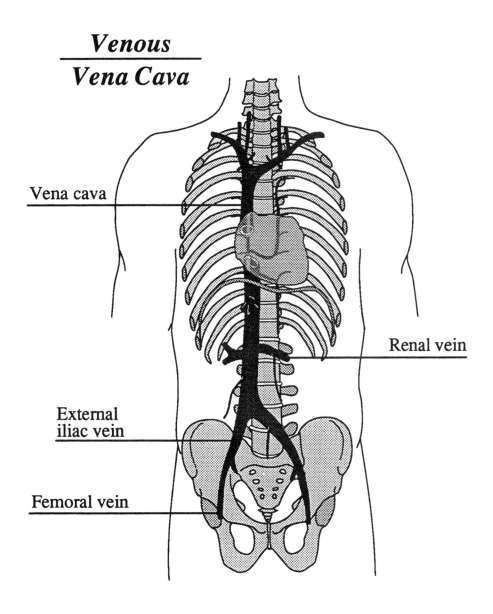

Venous
Vena Cava

Vena cava

Renal vein

External
iliac vein

Femoral vein

Anterior Heart

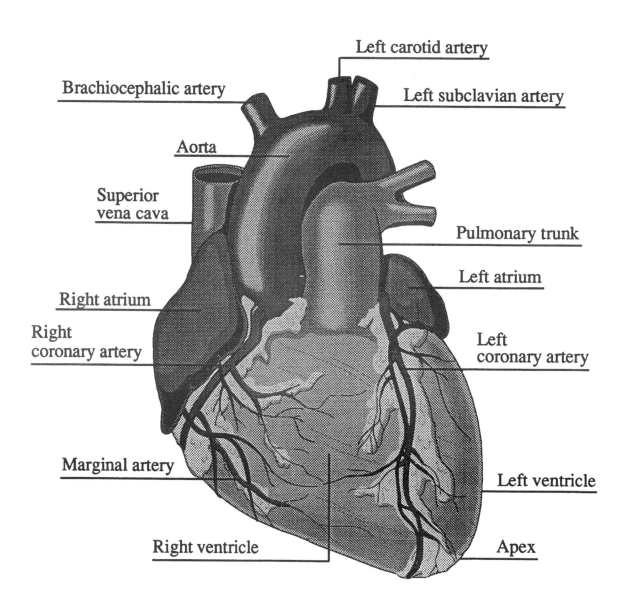

Left carotid artery

Brachiocephalic artery

Left subclavian artery

Aorta

Superior
vena cava

Pulmonary trunk

Left atrium

Right atrium

Right
coronary artery

Left
coronary artery

Marginal artery

Left ventricle

Right ventricle

Apex

"LifeART Images Copyright © 1991 by TechPool Studios, Inc."

Posterior Heart

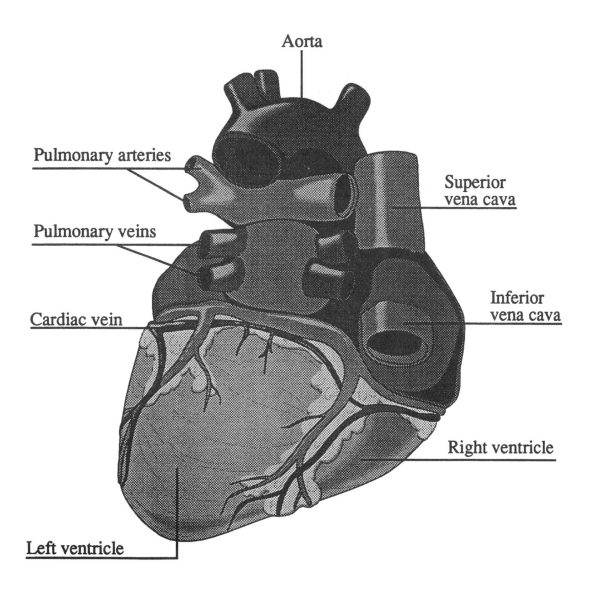

Aorta

Pulmonary arteries

Superior
vena cava

Pulmonary veins

Cardiac vein

Inferior
vena cava

Right ventricle

Left ventricle

Internal Heart

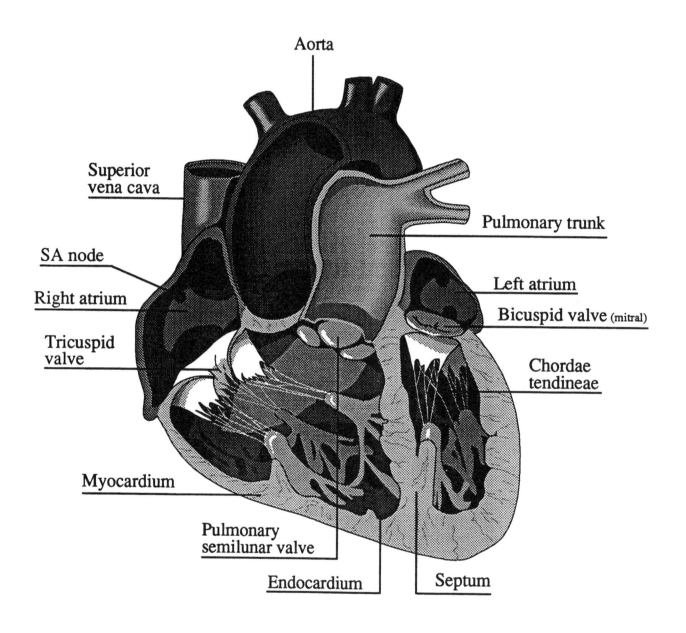

Aorta

Superior
vena cava

Pulmonary trunk

SA node

Left atrium

Right atrium

Bicuspid valve (mitral)

Tricuspid
valve

Chordae
tendineae

Myocardium

Pulmonary
semilunar valve

Endocardium

Septum

Pumping Action of the Heart

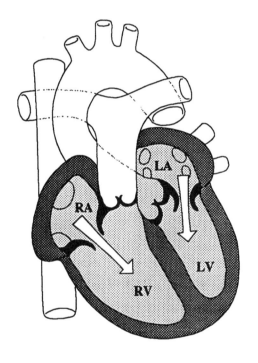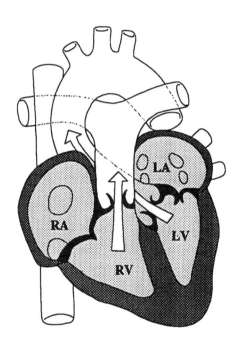

Open Book Quiz:

Name: Kim Dabacon

Session: 6

1. What is: COPD...CHD...MI?

    COPD- chronic obstructive pulmonary disease.
    CHD-coronary Heart Disease
    MI- myocardial Infarction

2. What two substances do the alveoli exchange in the blood?

    Oxygen + carbon Dioxide in the blood.

3. Name three types of blood cells.

    Red blood cells
    white blood cells
    Platelets

4. What does the pericardium do?

    Is a membranous bag that holds the heart.

5. Where is the aorta? What does it do?

    The aorta is in the left Ventricle + it carries
    the oxygenated blood to the body.

6. Explain systolic and diastolic.

    Systolic - is a measurement of the bloods pressure
    against artery walls when the Heart works.
    Diastolic- measurement of bloodPressure during the
    hearts Relaxation period.

7. What is angina?

    Discomfort or pain the in chest that is usually
    Relieved by Rest.

8. Describe atherosclerosis.

    Causes a narrowing of interior portions of arteries.
    The narrowing occurs in Relation to the accumulation
    of lipids + other substances on the inner wall
    of the blood vessel.

Medical Basics

TOPIC: DIGESTIVE SYSTEM

Roots:
hepato	= liver
gastro	= stomach
enter	= intestine
lapar	= abdomen
procto	= rectum

1. Other names for the digestive system are the gastrointestinal or GI system, and the **alimentary tract** or **alimentary canal.** The alimentary canal has several accessory organs that assist in this process. This system is involved with the ingestion, digestion, absorption, and elimination of food and food products.

2. The process begins as food enters the mouth, and is completed when the undigested waste is expelled through the rectum and anus as feces.

3. Food moves through the digestive system by muscular, wave-like contractions, called **peristalsis.**

4. Food takes 10-20 hours to pass through the body.

5. The mouth, teeth, tongue, and salivary glands first begin to process the food. When swallowed, the food continues through the:

Esophagus ....A straight, collapsible tube, behind the trachea.

The Stomach ....is a J-shaped pouch, hanging under the diaphragm. It connects with the esophagus at the top. It secretes gastric juices containing hydrochloric acid and digestive enzymes. The pyloric sphincter separates the stomach from the small intestines. When the sphincter closes, food remains in the stomach. When the sphincter opens the stomach contents are allowed to enter the small intestines.

The small intestine ....is 20-30 feet long, and 1 inch in diameter. It is composed of the duodenum (10 inch), Jejunum (8 feet), and the ileum (12 feet)

Function: Completes digestion, absorbs the end products into the blood stream. At the distal end of the ileum the ileo-cecal valve separates the small intestines from the large intestine.

TOPIC: DIGESTIVE SYSTEM   (Continued)

The large intestine ....is 5-6 feet long, 2 1/2 inches in diameter. It consists of the cecum, the colon, the rectum, and the anal canal. The appendix is located in the cecum. The colon is divided into 4 portions: the ascending, transverse, descending, and sigmoid colon. The rectum lies next to the sacrum. It ends about 5 centimeters below the tip of the coccyx, where it becomes the anal canal. Function: absorption of water and elimination of waste.

TOPIC: ACCESSORY ORGANS TO THE DIGESTIVE SYSTEM

1. **The Pancreas** is a gland directly behind the stomach, between the spleen and the duodenum. The pancreas:

   Connects to the duodenum by the pancreatic duct.

   Secretes enzymes capable of digesting carbohydrates, fats, proteins, and nucleic acids.

   Produces insulin. Insulin is responsible for the absorption of glucose into cells.

2. **The Liver** is the largest gland in the body, weighing 3-4 lbs. in the adult. It is located just below the diaphragm. It is one of the body's most vital organs. The liver functions to:

   Store and filter blood.

   Secrete bile (1 pint daily).

   Convert sugars into glycogen.

The cells in the liver are microscopic, but they can do many things at once. They enable the liver to perform the duties of:

a factory ....producing chemical compounds.

a warehouse ....storing glycogen, iron and vitamins A,D,B12.

a waste disposal plant ....excreting bile pigments, urea, and detoxicants. It removes damaged red blood cells and foreign substances by phagocytosis. It alters the composition of toxic substances, like alcohol.

a power plant ....breaking down complex substances, with the release of energy as a byproduct.

The fuel of the body is a simple sugar called glucose. It is converted into glycogen. The liver stores glycogen for future use.

TOPIC: DIGESTIVE SYSTEM   (Continued)

3. Severe liver damage can be caused by many things. A few of them are:

    Carbon tetrachloride fume inhalation.

    Acetaminophen overdosage (tylenol).

4. **Cirrhosis** of the liver is a disease characterized by loss of functioning liver cells, and a increased resistance to the flow of blood through the liver. There are several types of cirrhosis:

    alcoholic ....Approximately 20 percent of alcoholics develop cirrhosis.

    biliary ....obstruction of the bile duct, resulting in jaundice (jaundice = excess bilirubin in the blood causes bile pigments to be stored in various tissue, resulting in a yellow appearance)

    toxic ....from poisoning by carbon tetrachloride.

5. **Hepatitis** is an inflammation of the liver. It can be caused by a viral infection, or the presence of toxins. Hepatitis can be secondary to things like mononucleoses or cirrhosis. Medications such as INH (isoniazid given for Tuberculosis), NSAIDS (nonsteroidal antiinflammatory drugs such as Advil, Feldene, Naprosyn), or steroids (prednisone, cortisone,) can cause inflammation of the liver.

6. **The Gallbladder** is a small, pear shaped sac located under the liver. It is attached to the liver by fibrous tissue. Bile produced by the liver passes to the gallbladder through a small tube called the cystic duct. This duct branches off from the bile duct. The bile duct carries bile from the liver to the duodenum. The gallbladder stores the bile until it is needed to emulsify fats contained in food.

    Gallstones can form in this system when there's a problem with the chemical composition of the bile. That can happen when the bile is overloaded with cholesterol. The most common type of gallstone is composed of cholesterol. Removal of the gallstones, or the gallbladder has shown no long term complications.

7. **Cholecystitis** is inflammation of the gallbladder. **Cholecystectomy** is removal of the gallbladder.

8. **Diabetes mellitus** is a condition characterized by a high blood glucose level and the appearance of glucose in the urine due to a deficiency of insulin. The amount of blood sugar rises, causing the kidneys to excrete the extra sugar. This causes the production of excessive amounts of urine. This creates two of the major symptoms of uncontrolled diabetes: excessive urination, and dehydration.

TOPIC: DIGESTIVE SYSTEM   (Continued)

Diabetes mellitus:

type I ....insulin dependent..(IDDM) usually has it's onset before age 20. It is an autoimmune disease in which the body's immune system destroys the cells in the pancreas, so that the ability to secrete insulin is diminished.

type II ....non insulin dependent..(NIDDM) is found in 70-80 percent of diabetic patients. Usually appears gradually after age 40, and produces milder symptoms than type I.

Diabetes can produce many ongoing problems for the individual. Wounds may not heal as quickly as they would in the individual without diabetes.

Diabetic retinopathy ....problems with the blood vessels in the retina of the eye.

Neuropathy ....damage to nerve fibers (polyneuropathy = many nerves damaged, peripheral neuropathy = nerves in hands or feet damaged)

Atherosclerosis and high blood pressure ....have a higher than average incidence in diabetics.

TOPIC: OTHER PROBLEMS OF THE DIGESTIVE SYSTEM

1. **Esophagus:**

   esophageal diverticulum...............Small area of outpouching tissue.usually at top end of esophagus.

   esophageal varices ....Enlarged veins at lower end of esophagus.

2. **Gastric Ulcer:** A raw, open area on the inner wall of the stomach.

3. **Gastritis:** Inflammation of the lining of the stomach, causing nausea and vomiting.

   Gastroenteritis: Sudden inflammation of stomach and intestine, causing diarrhea and vomiting. Symptoms usually subside in 36-48 hours.

4. **Peptic ulcer:** A ulcer that may occur in the esophagus, stomach, or duodenum.

   They are the most common in the first part of the duodenum or lower part of the stomach. Acid is produced in the stomach. In the presence of an irritant, such as alcohol, bile, bacteria, caffeine, medications (aspirin), the acid may work through the protective lining, creating a ulceration.

   Symptoms can include pain, nausea, loss of appetite. If the ulceration continues to grow, it may involve a blood vessel, causing bleeding. If it continues to grow it may perforate..or eat through the tissue completely. Treatment can include medication, diet, and/or surgery.

5. **Gastrectomy:** Removal of a portion of the stomach. A total gastrectomy is rarely done.

6. **Gastroenterologist:** A physician (MD) specializing in problems of the digestive system.

7. **Vagotomy:** The vagus nerve controls the production of digestive acid. It can be surgically cut as a method of treating a peptic ulcer.

8. **Paralytic ileus:** A failure of the normal contractility of the muscles of the intestine...usually temporary. Peristalsis stops. It can follow abdominal surgery or can be induced by severe abdominal injury.

9. **Colostomy:** Surgical opening of some portion of the colon to the abdominal surface.

TOPIC: DIAGNOSING G.I. CONDITIONS

1. **Barium swallow** - used to diagnose a problem in the upper GI. The barium is impervious to X-Ray. The patient swallows the barium, and X-rays are taken.

2. **Barium Enema** - used to diagnose problems in the lower GI.

3. A **stool sample** - will identify blood in the stool.

4. **CBC** (complete blood count) - if a person is anemic, it may indicate bleeding somewhere in the GI system.

5. **Liver enzymes** - will indicate liver damage.

6. **Blood sugar** - indicates the blood's sugar level.

7. **Sed Rate** (sedimentation rate) - decreased in liver disease - increased with infection.

8 **Sigmoidoscopy** - the interior of the sigmoid colon is visualized by the physician with the aid of a sigmoidoscope.

ICD-9 Codes commonly seen for the digestive system:

789.0....................Abdominal pain

531.90 ....Ulcers/Gastric

TOPIC: STRESS

1. Examples:

stress fracture ....a fracture, usually a hairline fracture, that develops gradually, in response to repeated and prolonged stress.

stress ulcer ....a peptic ulcer caused by acute or chronic stress such as cerebral trauma, burns, surgery, or acute infections

stress test ....a diagnostic test to evaluate cardiovascular function when the body is subjected to steadily increasing levels of work.

POST TRAUMATIC STRESS (PTS) ....stress following trauma. Diagnosis (DX): adjustment disorder, with anxious mood. The acute form has an onset of symptoms within six months of the trauma, with symptoms lasting less than six months. More than six months and it becomes chronic/delayed. (adjustment disorder, with anxious mood-symptoms such as nervousness, worry and jitteriness...ICD-9 309.24)

3. **Stress can lead to a major depressive disorder**...loss of interest in all or almost all usual activities and pastimes. The mood is characterized by the patients complaints of feeling: depressed, sad, blue, hopeless, low down in the dumps, irritable. These feelings must be predominant and relatively persistent to be classified as a major depressive disorder. ICD-9...296.30

4. **Anxiety** produces a feeling of apprehension, worry, or dread. It's a normal reaction to something that threatens the body, lifestyle, values, or loved ones. Excessive anxiety can interfere with efficient functioning of the individual.

anxiety disorders.......................a group of psychiatric disorders that include phobia's, panic, obsessive compulsive behavior, and anxiety.

anxiety neurosis ....a mental disorder characterized by excessive anxiety. May be manifested when an individual without organic disease complains of palpitation, heart pain, dyspepsia, constriction of the throat, bandlike pressure around the head, or cold, sweaty tremulous extremities. ICD-9...300.00

TOPIC: STRESS (Continued)

5. **Adjustment Reaction** - is also called adjustment disorder. A non adaptive reaction to an identifiable source of stress, that occurs within three months of the onset of the stress. It is assumed that the problem will eventually stop when the source of stress is removed. ICD-9...309.28

6. **Drug dependence** - also called substance use disorder. The inability to cut down on, or stop the daily use of any of the following: alcohol, prescription and non prescription drugs, tobacco. It is characterized by behavioral changes that include a compulsion to take the drug on a continuous basis in order to experience it's psychic effects, or to avoid the discomfort of it's absence. ICD-9...304.10

7. The **MMPI** is a baseline test given for psychiatric diagnoses.

8. The **DSM III** is the Diagnostic and Statistical Manual of Mental Disorders, Third Edition. This text is used as a guideline for the diagnostic interpretation of the MMPI, and for rating mental illness.

9. Mental illness ratings are clearly outlined in 436-35-400.

TOPIC: MEDICATIONS

1. There are 5 classes of medications frequently seen in Workers' Compensation

    1. Analgesics

    2. Anti-inflammatory Agents

    3. Muscle relaxants

    4. Anti-ulcer agents

    5. Anti-anxiety agents

1. **Analgesics:** These medications are given for pain. They are given a classification of 1 to 4, with one being the most addictive. The classifications are also referred to as schedules.

    Examples:

    #1...Heroin

    #2...Percocet, Percodan, Tylox, Codeine, Morphine, Hydrocodone

    #3...Vicodin, Phenaphen with Codeine, Talacen, Talwin NX, Wygesic

    #4...Pentazocine, Propoxyphene

    A. Darvon is a mild narcotic, related in chemical structure to methadone. When used, the use of alcohol, other analgesics, or tranquilizers needs to be monitored, as they potentiate the effect of the medication.

    B. Tylenol is a brand of acetaminophen. It is metabolized in the liver, and excreted through the kidneys. A few medications containing Tylenol are Darvocet-N, Percocet, Phenaphen w/Codeine, Talacen, Tylenol w/Codeine, Vicodin, Wygesic.

    C. Drug interactions:

    Valium ....taken with one of the analgesic pain meds will increase drowsiness.

    Elavil ....taken with one of the analgesic pain meds will increase sedation.

    Nardil, Parnate, Marplan ......taken with analgesic pain meds are potentially fatal. These medications remain in the body up to 14 days.

TOPIC: MEDICATIONS (Continued)

2. **Anti-inflammatory Agents** (NSAIDS-nonsteroidal anti-inflammatory drugs): These medications are **site specific.** A damaged muscle gives off **prostaglandin.** NSAID's are anti-prostaglandin medications. When the tablet is taken, the medication does not work on the whole body. It works only on the area giving off the prostaglandin.

    A. NSAIDS should be taken with food. Adverse reactions include stomach irritation, ulcer, and decreased kidney function.

    B. Examples of NSAIDS are: Ansaid, Feldene, Indocine, Motrin, Naprosyn, Voltarin, Aspirin.

3. **Muscle relaxants:** These medications reduce local pain and tenderness, but are nonspecific to site. They effect the whole body.

    A. Flexeril is closely related to Elavil (an antidepressant).

    B. Lioresal is the muscle relaxant of choice with spinal cord injuries.

    C. Norflex should not be given to workers with blurred vision, glaucoma, or urinary retention.

4. **Anti-ulcer Agents:**

    A. Prevents the ulcer from forming: Cytotec

    B. GI barrier (Like Pepto-Bismol coats the lining): Carafate

    C. Decreases stomach secretion: Tagamet, Zantac, Axid, Pepcid

    D. Inhibits gastric secretion: Prilosec

5. **Anti-anxiety agents:** Class 4 controlled substances. They include tranquilizers, sedatives, antihistamines, and hypnotics.

    A. **Tranquilizer:** Atavan, Librium, Serax, Tranxene, Valium, Xanax

    B. **Sedative:** Restoril, Centrax, Dalmane

    C. **Hypnotic:** Halcion, given at bedtime, maximum dosage is .25 mg one time daily.

    D. Drug interactions:

        1. Tagamet and Darvocet-N 100 will increase the effect of the anti-anxiety agents.

        2. Taken with alcohol, they increase drowsiness and cause dizziness.

Digestive System

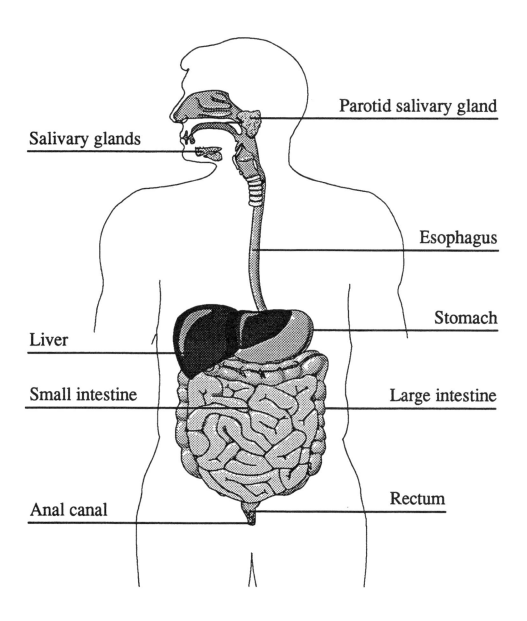

Parotid salivary gland

Salivary glands

Esophagus

Stomach

Liver

Small intestine

Large intestine

Anal canal

Rectum

Stomach

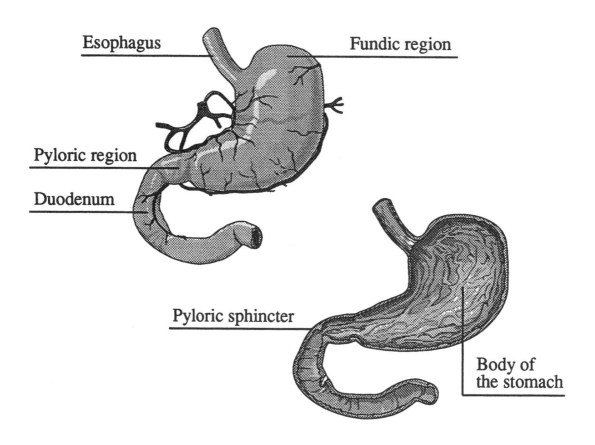

Esophagus

Fundic region

Pyloric region

Duodenum

Pyloric sphincter

Body of
the stomach

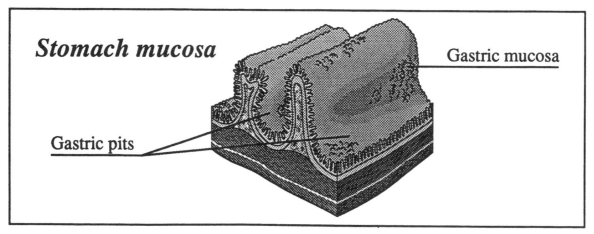

Stomach mucosa

Gastric mucosa

Gastric pits

"LifeART Images Copyright © 1991 by TechPool Studios, Inc."

Fig: 7-C

Accessory Organs to the Digestive System

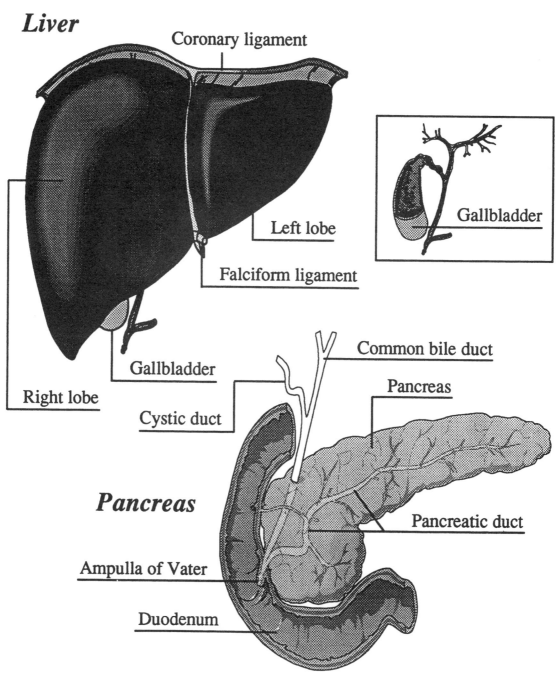

Liver

Coronary ligament

Left lobe

Falciform ligament

Gallblabber

Right lobe

Gallbladder

Cystic duct

Common bile duct

Pancreas

Pancreatic duct

Pancreas

Ampulla of Vater

Duodenum

Open Book Quiz:

Name: Kim Dabaen

Session: 7

1. Where is the esophagus? What does it do?

   A straight, collapsible tube, behind the trachea.
   Connects to the stomach—

2. What is the largest gland in the body? Give 2 of its functions.

   The Liver — 1. Store & filter blood.
   2. Secrete bile — 1 pint daily.
   3. Convert sugars into glycogen.

3. How is bilirubin related to jaundice?

   Excess bilirubin in the blood causes bile pigments
   to be stored in various tissue, resulting in jaundice
   a yellow appearance.

4. How is insulin related to type 1 and type II diabetes?

   Type I — Insulin dependent diabetes.

   Type II — non insulin dependent.

5. How are retinopathy and neuropathy related to diabetes?

   Retinopathy — problems with the blood vessels in the
   retina of the eye
   Neuropathy — damage to nerve fibers —

6. Why would a doctor recommend a vagotomy?

   The vagus nerve controls the production of
   digestive acid. It can be surgically cut as a method
   of treating a peptic ulcer.

7. What is a peptic ulcer? Where can it occur?
   — acid in the stomach — working thru the protective lining creating
   — a ulcer that may occur in the esophagus, stomach
   or duodenum.

8. Describe two ways anti-ulcer medications help a ulcer.

   1. Prevents the ulcer from forming: Cytotec

   2. Inhibits gastric secretion: Prilosec.

9. How does anti-inflammatory medication work?

   There site specific they work only in the areas
   giving off prostaglandin.

10. What is Prostaglandin?

   a damaged muscle gives off prostaglandin —

127

Bibliography

Bender, Matthew, Attorney's Textbook of Medicine: Manual of Traumatic Injuries, Matthew Bender, 1962.

Chabner, Davi-Ellen, The Language of Medicine, W.B. Saunders Company, Philadelphia, PA, 1991.

DePalma, Rothman, The Intervertebral Disc, Thiene Medical Publishers, New York, 1990.

Hole, John W., Human Anatomy and Physiology, Wm. C. Brown Publishing, Iowa, 1990.

Levy, Barry, David Wegman, Occupational Health, Recognizing and Preventing Work-Related Disease, Little, Brown and Company, Boston/Toronto, 1988.

Rockwood & Matsen, The Shoulder, Volumes 1 & 11, W.B. Saunders Company, Philadelphia, PA, 1975.

Roy, Steven, Richard Irvin, Sports Medicine, Prentice - Hall, New Jersey, 1983.

Tierney, Lawrence M., Current Medical Diagnosis & Treatment 1995, Appleton & Lang, Norwalk, Connecticut, 1995.

Turek, Orthopaedics Principals and their Application, J.B. Lippincott Company, 1977.

Warwick, Williams, Gray's Anatomy, Gramercy Books, New York, 1977.

130

Congratulations on your completion of Medical Basics

Awarded to

Kim Dabacon

Date: 1-9-2001

Linda Gifford-Meuleveld, R.N., COHN-S
Medical Training Coordinator

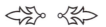

HOW MUCH HAVE YOU LEARNED?

(4 POINTS EACH)

1. What is the difference between conductive and perceptive impairment?

2. What is cephalgia?

3. Name the joint often abbreviated as "TMJ".

4. Name three types of cumulative problems that can result in TMJ.

5. What is the rotator cuff?

6. What two diagnostic tests are useful in diagnosing a rotator cuff tear?

7. Name two symptoms of adhesive capsulitis.

8. List four facts about carpal tunnel syndrome.

9. How is an indirect inguinal hernia different from a hiatal hernia?

10. What can cause bursitis?

11. Name a synovial joint that is frequently injured.

12. Why would a physician do an arthroscopy?

13. Name (1) muscle in the upper back and (1) muscle in the lower back that are often involved

in a back strain.

14. What vertebrae are most commonly injured?

15. Describe radiculitis.

16. What is sciatica?

17. What is a laminectomy?

18. What happens when a disk herniates?

19. Name 4 knee ligaments.

20. What is the medical name for the kneecap?

21. What is the purpose of the two menisci in each knee joint?

22. Chondromalacia affects what part of the knee?

23. Name two NSAIDS.

24. How do they work in the body?

25. Why would a physician order Flexeril for an injured worker?

EXTRA CREDIT: You may choose 1 or 2...and earn up to five extra credit points for each. I will

judge how many points to give according to the completeness of your answer.

1. How do medications like Tagamet, Zantec and Pepcid act in the body?

2. Describe Hepatitis B.

3. A worker has been admitted to the hospital with dyspnea and atelectasis. What does that

tell you?

4. An injured worker has type 1 diabetes mellitus. Describe one ongoing problem the worker

may encounter with this type of diabetes.